Biology and Management of Lung Cancer

Cancer Treatment and Research

WILLIAM L. MCGUIRE, *series editor*

1. R.B. Livingston, ed., Lung Cancer 1. 1981. ISBN 90-247-2394-9.
2. G.B. Humphrey, L.P. Dehner, G.B. Grindey and R.T. Acton, eds., Pediatric Oncology 1. 1981. ISBN 90-247-2408-2.
3. J.J. DeCosse and P. Sherlock, eds., Gastrointestinal Cancer 1. 1981. ISBN 90-247-2461-9.
4. J.M. Bennett, ed., Lymphomas 1. 1981. ISBN 90-247-2479-1.
5. C.D. Bloomfield, ed., Adult Leukemias 1. 1982. ISBN 90-247-2478-3.
6. D.F. Paulson, Genitourinary Cancer 1. 1982. ISBN 90-247-2480-5.
7. F.M. Muggia, ed., Cancer Chemotherapy 1. 1982. ISBN 90-247-2713-8.
8. G.B. Humphrey and G.B. Grindley, Pediatric Oncology 2. 1982. ISBN 90-247-2702-2.
9. John J. Costanzi, ed., Malignant Melanoma 1. 1982. ISBN 90-247-2706-5.
10. C.T. Griffiths, A.F. Fuller, ed., Gynecologic Oncology. 1983. ISBN 90-247-2753-7

Biology and Management of Lung Cancer

edited by

F. ANTHONY GRECO

Department of Medicine, Vanderbilt University Medical Center,Nashville, Tennessee, USA

1983 **MARTINUS NIJHOFF PUBLISHERS**
a member of the KLUWER ACADEMIC PUBLISHERS GROUP
BOSTON / THE HAGUE / DORDRECHT / LANCASTER

IV

Distributors

for the United States and Canada: Kluwer Boston, Inc., 190 Old Derby Street, Hingham, MA 02043, USA
for all other countries: Kluwer Academic Publishers Group, Distribution Center, P.O.Box 322, 3300 AH Dordrecht, The Netherlands

Library of Congress Cataloging in Publication Data

```
Main entry under title:

Biology and management of lung cancer.

   (Cancer treatment and research ; v. 11)
   1. Lungs--Cancer.  I. Greco, F. Anthony (Frank
Anthony), 1947-    .  II. Series.  [DNLM:
1. Lung neoplasms.  Wl CA693 v.11 / WF 658 B615]
RC280.L8B54  1983      616.99'424      82-14489
```

ISBN 0-89838-554-7

Contents

Foreword to the series

Where do you begin to look for a recent, authoritative article on the diagnosis or management of a particular malignancy? The few general oncology textbooks are generally out of date. Single papers in specialized journals are informative but seldom comprehensive; these are more often preliminary reports on a very limited number of patients. Certain general journals frequently publish good indepth reviews of cancer topics, and published symposium lectures are often the best overviews available. Unfortunately, these reviews and supplements appear sporadically, and the reader can never be sure when a topic of special interest will be covered.

Cancer Treatment and Research is a series of authoritative volumes which aim to meet this need. It is an attempt to establish a critical mass of oncology literature covering virtually all oncology topics, revised frequently to keep the coverage up to date, easily available on a single library shelf or by a single personal subscription.

We have approached the problem in the following fashion. First, by dividing the oncology literature into specific subdivisions such as lung cancer, genitourinary cancer, pediatric oncology, etc. Second, by asking eminent authorities in each of these areas to edit a volume on the specific topic on an annual or biannual basis. Each topic and tumor type is covered in a volume appearing frequently and predictably, discussing current diagnosis, staging, markers, all forms of treatment modalities, basic biology, and more.

In *Cancer Treatment and Research,* we have an outstanding group of editors, each having made a major commitment to bring to this new series the very best literature in his or her field. Martinus Nijhoff Publishers has made an equally major commitment to the rapid publication of high quality books, and world-wide distribution.

Where can you go to find quickly a recent authoritative article on any major oncology problem? We hope that *Cancer Treatment and Research* provides an answer.

WILLIAM L. McGUIRE
Series Editor

Preface

Lung cancer remains an extremely difficult neoplasm to treat effectively. A large part of our lack of success in dealing with these patients is related to our empiric therapeutic attempts. Slowly our basic understanding of the lung cancers is improving and techniques are becoming available to allow us to better understand the biology of these neoplasms. This volume reviews several areas of interest in regard to the biologic behavior and characteristics of lung cancer.

Chapters deal with the *in vitro* growth of small cell lung cancer, the investigation of growth factors in human lung cancer, the production of monoclonal antibodies against lung cancer and the application and potential usefulness of the human tumor cloning assay in lung cancer management. These avenues of investigation are likely to establish a more scientific basis on which more rational therapy can be designed.

Carney and associates have established several continuous small cell lung cancer cell lines in their laboratory. The amine precursor uptake and decarboxylation (APUD) properties of this neoplasm have been confirmed by demonstrating the presence of neurosecretory granules and high levels of the APUD enzyme L-dopa decarboxylase. In addition, several new markers have been documented including bombesin, creatine-kinase BB and neuron-specific enolase. These tumor products along with others may be useful serum markers in patients with small cell lung cancer. *In vitro* growth requirements have also been identified in a serum-free chemical medium, the HITES medium. These studies may be close to finding growth inhibitors which are clinically applicable. Preliminary studies reported by Carney *et al.* also show what appears to be a specific cytogenetic abnormality in small cell lung cancer, a deletion involving chromosome 3 (3p). Such a marker, if confirmed, would not only help to better identify the neoplasm, but would be very helpful in various other studies by providing an accurate *in vitro* marker.

Sherwin and Todaro review their work with transforming growth factors, a class of peptide growth factors which are produced by lung cancer cells *in vitro*. It also appears that several patients with advanced cancers, including lung cancer, have detectable tumor-associated transforming growth factors in their urine. The concept of 'autocrine secretion' (the secretion of growth factors such as transforming growth factors and often related molecules by tumor cells required for tumor growth and survival *in vivo*) forms the basis for attempts to manipulate these substances in hopes of preventing or inhibiting tumor growth.

Cuttitta and associates discuss their work on the generation and characterization of monoclonal antibodies directed against human lung cancer. Details are reviewed regarding small cell lung cancer antibodies which preferentially bind to tissue culture cell lines and autopsy tissue samples, but not with a variety of autologous cell lines and normal tissues. Although the specific antigen or antigens are not yet identified, several monoclonal antibodies have been used to immunohistochemically stain patients' tumors, to type human tumors and to define various antigenic determinates of small cell lung cancer. The potential of the specific binding properties of monoclonal antibodies may form the basis of useful therapies. Conjugation of antibodies to drugs, radioisotopes or toxic molecules offers the potential for the 'magic bullet'.

Callahan *et al.* review the limitations, applications and potential usefulness of the tumor cloning assay in lung cancer management. The current clinical usefulness is limited by the relatively low growth rate (50%), the time and expense involved and the low plating efficiency even when there is growth. Only a small number of drugs can be tested against most individual tumors since the plating efficiency is often low, and the results obtained take about two weeks. However, the system is being refined and of those tumors with adequate growth the prediction of *in vivo* tumor response has been good, particularly for predicting drug resistance. Although the determination of *in vitro* drug sensitivity appears to be in the 'infancy period', it will continue to grow and develop.

Other contributors to this volume deal with the problem of accurate histologic diagnosis in poorly differentiated lung cancers, the riddle of cachexia associated with lung cancer, the morphologic alterations of small cell lung cancer following intensive therapy, and the promise of the neurophysins as reliable biochemical small cell lung cancer markers.

Two novel and potentially useful therapeutic strategies are reviewed: the use of adjuvant surgery in patients with limited stage small cell lung cancer and the use of high-dose chemotherapy with autologous bone marrow transplantation. Finally, a comprehensive review of therapeutic attempts in advanced non-small cell lung cancer is presented.

The majority of the work presented in this volume deals with new areas of clinical and basic research of the lung cancer problem. The contributors to this volume represent a small number of the many interested investigators who will eventually help to find the necessary answers.

F. ANTHONY GRECO

List of Contributors

BLOCK, Jerome B., M.D., University of California, Los Angeles School of Medicine, Department of Medicine, Harbor-UCLA Medical Center, Division of Medical Oncology, Torrance, CA 90509, USA.

CALLAHAN, S. Kent, M.D., Department of Medicine, University of Texas, Health Science Center, San Antonio, TX 78284, USA.

CARNEY, Desmond N., M.D., NCI-Naval Medical Oncology Branch, National Naval Medical Center, Bethesda, MD 20814, USA.

CHLEBOWSKI, Rowan T., M.D., Ph.D., University of California, Los Angeles School of Medicine, Department of Medicine, Harbor-UCLA Medical Center, Division of Medical Oncology, Torrance, CA 90509, USA.

COLTMAN, Charles A. Jr., Department of Medicine, University of Texas Health Science Center, San Antonio, TX 78284, USA.

COMIS, Robert L., M.D., Associate Professor of Medicine, Chief, Section of Medical Oncology, Department of Medicine, State University of New York, Upstate Medical Center, 750 East Adams Street, Syracuse, NY 13210, USA.

CUTTITTA, Frank, M.D., NCI-Naval Medical Oncology Branch (DCT/NCI/NIH) and Litton Bionetics, National Naval Medical Center, Bethesda, MD 20814, USA.

FER, Mehmet F., M.D., Assistant Professor, Department of Medicine, Division of Oncology, Vanderbilt University Medical Center, Nashville, TN 37232, USA.

GAZDAR, Adi F., M.D., NCI-Naval Medical Oncology Branch (DCT/NCI/NIH) National Naval Medical Center, Bethesda, MD 20814, USA.

GRECO, F. Anthony, M.D., Associate Professor, Department of Medicine, Director, Division of Oncology, Vanderbilt University Medical Center, Nashville, TN 37232, USA.

GROSH, William W., M.D., Research Fellow, Department of Medicine,

Division of Oncology, Vanderbilt University Medical Center, Nashville, TN 37232, USA.

HANDE, Kenneth R., M.D., Nashville Veterans Administration Medical Center and Division Medical Oncology, Vanderbilt University School of Medicine, Nashville, TN 37232, USA.

HEBER, David, M.D., Ph.D., University of California, Los Angeles School of Medicine, Department of Medicine, Harbor-UCLA Medical Center, Divisions of Endocrinology and Metabolism, Torrance, CA 90509, USA.

KITTEN, Cliff, M.D., Department of Medicine, University of Texas Health Science Center, San Antonio, TX 78284, USA.

LUKEMAN, John M., M.D., The University of Texas System Cancer Center, M.D. Anderson Hospital and Tumor Institute, Department of Pathology, Houston, TX 77030, USA.

MACKAY, Bruce, M.D., Ph.D., The University of Texas System Cancer Center, M.D. Anderson Hospital and Tumor Institute, Department of Pathology, Houston, TX 77030, USA.

MALCOLM, Arnold W., M.D., Nashville Veterans Administration Medical Center and Division of Radiology, Vanderbilt University School of Medicine, Nashville, TN 37232, USA.

MAURER, L. Herbert, M.D., Department of Medicine, Dartmouth Medical School, Hanover, NH 03755, USA.

MINNA, John D., M.D., NCI-Naval Medical Oncology Branch (DCT/NCI/NIH) National Naval Medical Center, Bethesda, MD 20814, USA.

NORTH, William G., M.D., Department of Physiology, Dartmouth Medical School, Hanover, NH 03755, USA.

O'DONNELL, Joseph F., M.D., Department of Medicine, Dartmouth Medical School, Hanover, NH 03755, USA.

OIE, Herbert K., M.D., NCI-Naval Medical Oncology Branch (DCT/NCI/NIH) and Litton Bionetics, National Naval Medical Center, Bethesda, MD 20814, USA.

ROSEN, Steven, M.D., NCI-Naval Medical Oncology Branch, National Naval Medical Center, Bethesda, MD 20814, USA.

SHERWIN, Stephen A., M.D., Biological Response Modifiers Program, National Cancer Institute, Frederick, MD 21701, USA.

TODARO, George J., M.D., Laboratory of Viral Carcinogenesis, National Cancer Institute, Frederick, MD 21701, USA.

VON HOFF, Daniel D., M.D., Department of Medicine, University of Texas Health Science Center, San Antonio, TX 78284, USA.

WOLFF, Steven N., M.D., Division of Oncology, Department of Medicine, Vanderbilt University Medical Center, Nashville, TN 37232, USA.

1. The *In Vitro* Growth and Characterization of Small Cell Lung Cancer

DESMOND N. CARNEY, ADI F. GAZDAR, HERBERT K. OIE, FRANCIS CUTTITTA
and JOHN D. MINNA

1. INTRODUCTION

Recent statistics concerning the incidence of lung cancer have demonstrated an increase in the number of new cases and the number of deaths for this disease among the population of the USA [1]. In 1981, an estimated 115,000 people will develop this disease. There are four major histologic types of lung cancer: epidermoid (or squamous) lung cancer, adenocarcinoma, large cell carcinoma, and small cell lung cancer. Because of a number of biologic differences between small cell lung cancer (SCLC) (which accounts for 20–25 % of all cases) and the other varieties of lung cancer (the so-called non-small cell lung cancers, non-SCLC) including a more rapid tumor cell proliferation, a greater tendency for early regional and metastatic dissemination, and a greater sensitivity to both chemotherapy and radiation therapy [2–5], in therapeutic management, patients with SCLC are separated from those with non-SCLC. Unlike non-SCLC lung cancers, considerable advances have been made in the therapy of patients with SCLC. Using combination chemotherapy a clinical response will be achieved in 70–95 % of all patients, with approximately 40 % of patients achieving a complete remission. Unfortunately, responses are usually short, and median duration of survival for all patients is only 10.6 months [2]. Response to subsequent therapy following relapse is observed in only the minority of patients. However, although the vast majority of patients with SCLC will die of their disease, approximately 5–10 % of all patients will be cured.

The cell of origin of SCLC is considered to be the endocrine cell (Kultschitzkey cell) present in the normal respiratory mucosa which expresses a variety of APUD (amine precursor uptake and decarboxylation) properties. The recognition that SCLC was associated with a variety of paraneoplastic syndromes secondary to 'ectopic' hormone secretion and the recognition that SCLC cells contained neurosecretory granules lead to its inclusion in

Greco, FA (ed), Biology and Management of Lung Cancer. ISBN 0-89838-554-7.
© *1983, Martinus Nijhoff Publishers, Boston. Printed in The Netherlands.*

the APUD cell system of Pearse [6, 7]. To better understand the origin and biology of SCLC we, and others, have developed *in vitro* systems for supporting the continual growth of cell lines of SCLC obtained from patients with this disease. Several approaches have been utilized to develop these cell lines: (1) the direct culture in liquid medium (serum-supplemented medium, or selective chemically defined medium) of specimens obtained directly from patients, and (2) the establishment in culture of nude mouse SCLC heterotransplants developed by the inoculation of clinical material into these animals. Using these cell lines we have greatly expanded our understanding of the biology of SCLC. These lines have provided material for studying the origin and specific growth requirements of this tumor, and the mechanism of hormone synthesis and regulation of secretory products by this tumor. The cell lines provide a tool for the development of monoclonal antibodies with specificity for this tumor and also provide an *in vitro* model for the screening of new cytotoxic agents with potential clinical activity in small cell lung cancer. The use of cell lines of SCLC has permitted the identification of a specific cytogenetic abnormality not found in other types of lung cancer, or in other human tumors. All of these have direct application to patient management and treatment.

2. THE PRIMARY GROWTH AND *IN VITRO* CHARACTERISTICS OF SMALL CELL LUNG CANCER

Since the late 1970s, several laboratories have been successful in the establishment of continuous cell lines of SCLC [8–11]. While few have been cultured from primary tumors, cell lines have been cultured from a variety of metastatic sites. Although most specimens have been cultured from living patients, cell lines have been successfully established from autopsy specimens. Cell lines have been cultured from newly diagnosed, previously untreated patients and from patients who have relapsed from prior intensive combination chemotherapy, with or without radiation therapy. Although earlier attempts to establish cell lines of this tumor met with limited success, with improved techniques and better culture conditions cell lines can now be established from 50–75 % of all adequate specimens received in the laboratory. Two 'growth conditions' have improved our results: (1) the use of condition media from established cell lines of SCLC, greatly enhancing our ability to establish new cell lines [8] and suggesting that these tumors produce 'autostimulating' factors for the growth of SCLC cells, and (2) the use of a chemically defined, serum-free medium for SCLC (vide infra) [12].

For most cell lines the base medium used has been either RPMI 1640 medium (GIBCO, New York) or Waymouths MB 7521 medium [8, 9]. In

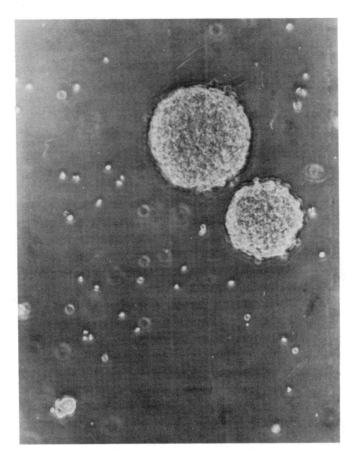

Figure 1. Classic morphological *in vitro* appearance of a cell line of SCLC NCI H378. The cells grow in tight spherical aggregates in suspension culture.

these media, once established as independent cell cultures, free of fibroblast or other stromal cell contamination, the tumor cells grow either as floating cell aggregates or as attached to substrate. In the latter cases, usually observed in Waymouths medium, as cell density increases, large clumps of cells detach from the surface of the dish and float [9]. A typical morphological appearance of SCLC culture is demonstrated in Figure 1.

In continuous culture, cell lines of SCLC have a relatively prolonged doubling time (49–96+ hours), express human isozymes, form colonies in soft agarose at an efficiency of 1–5%, and form tumors in athymic nude mice with the typical morphological characteristics of SCLC. The cells in culture have the typical cytological characteristics of SCLC of the intermediate cell type. Continuous cell lines of SCLC also express many APUD cell properties including neurosecretory granules, which may be present either singly,

4

Table 1. In vitro properties of established cell lines of small cell and non-small cell lung cancer

Test	Small cell	Non-small cell
Morphology	Floaters	Adherent
Nude mouse tumorigenicity	Yes	Yes
Neurosecretroy granules	Present	Absent
L-dopa decarboxylase	Elevated	Low/absent
Creatine-kinase BB	Elevated	Low/absent
Bombesin	Elevated	Absent
Neuron-specific enolase	Elevated	Low/absent
Deletion 3p	Present	Absent

or in clusters, and formaldehyde-induced fluorescence [8–12]. The key APUD enzyme, L-dopa decarboxylase (E.C. 1.1.28) (DDC), has been demonstrated in both clinical specimens, cell lines and nude mouse tumors of SCLC [13, 14]. While considerable heterogeneity of expression of this enzyme has been found in SCLC clinical specimens obtained from autopsy, ranging from absence of L-dopa decarboxylase activity in all lesions for some patients to low levels of the marker in metastatic sites in others, to full expression of APUD properties in all tumor lesions in others, values in patients with SCLC are considerably higher than values observed in tumor specimens obtained from patients with other forms of lung cancers (Table 1) [13–15]. Among cell lines of lung cancer, L-dopa decarboxylase activity clearly differentiates cell lines of SCLC origin from those of other cell types. Values in SCLC cell lines are almost 300-fold greater than those observed in a variety of other cell lung cancer cell lines [15]. Measurement of L-dopa decarboxylase activity also serves as a useful means for monitoring the process of 'transformation' of SCLC cells from typical SCLC to cells with other lung cancer morphology *in vivo* and *in vitro*. While clinical correlates of this transformation have been observed [16, 17], recent evidence suggests that this transformation, with loss of APUD cell properties, may be associated with an increased resistance to cytotoxic modalities (vide infra). Clearly this would be of major significance in the care of these patients.

3. *IN VIVO* AND *IN VITRO* BIOLOGIC MARKERS OF SMALL CELL LUNG CANCER

Among solid human tumors, small cell lung cancer is the one most frequently associated with the presence of paraneoplastic syndromes. Both *in vivo* and *in vitro* production of a wide variety of hormones has been recognized in SCLC [18–28]. Many hormones have been demonstrated in these patients including calcitonin, CEA, ACTH, ADH, neurophysins, etc. Because of the association of hormone production with SCLC, investigators have attempted to use these hormones as markers for disease extent and activity in patients with SCLC. (For detailed review see Hansen [26].) Although a large number of studies have reported on the value of serum markers in patients with SCLC, there are conflicting data on their use in the management of patients with SCLC. Some studies have demonstrated an excellent correlation between disease extent and response to therapy, with serum levels of certain markers including CEA, calcitonin and neurophysin [20–22], while other studies, using the same markers, have failed to demonstrate a useful correlation [23–26]. In addition, none of these markers are either specific enough or sensitive enough to encourage either their use in the histologie typing of a lung cancer or to achieve widespread use in the staging and treatment of patients with SCLC. For most studies, routine clinical examination and staging procedures have provided similar clinical data.

In contrast to the '*in vivo*' clinical setting, recent studies have clearly demonstrated that certain markers are very useful in separating tumor cell lines *in vitro* of SCLC from cell lines of other histologic types of lung cancer. These markers include creatine-kinase BB, bombesin and neuron-specific enolase [29–35] (Table 1).

Creatine-kinase BB (CK-BB), the BB isozyme of creatine-kinase (E.C. 2.7.3.2) is normally found in large amounts only in striated muscle, brain, bladder and gastrointestinal tract [29]. Because of reports that elevated serum levels of CK-BB had been identified in a small number of patients with SCLC, we measured the levels of CK-BB in continuous cultures of SCLC. Like DDC, levels of CK-BB in SCLC cultures and fresh specimens were considerably higher than that observed in non-SCLC specimens (Table 1). Serum CK-BB was also measured in patients with SCLC. Preliminary results demonstrated that serum levels of CK-BB correlated with the extent of disease, and that sequential measurements of CK-BB demonstrated an excellent correlation with the observed clinical response. These data suggest that serum CK-BB determinations may be useful for monitoring response to therapy in patients with SCLC [32].

More recently we have evaluated two other markers more frequently found in high amounts of brain tissue: bombesin and neuron-specific enolase. Bombesin is a tetradecapeptide found in high amounts in brain, stomach, intestine and fetal lung [30]. A number of biological activities have been ascribed to bombesin including hyperglycemia, anorexia, hypothermia and brain-site dependent analgesia [30]. Measurement of intracellular bombesin in cell lines of lung cancer has revealed that only lung cancer cell lines of SCLC origin expressed high levels of bombesin, while it was not detectable in non-SCLC lung cancer cultures. Because bombesin is secreted by these cell lines, it may be possible to measure serum levels of bombesin and correlate results with disease activity. Preliminary data from a small number of patients has demonstrated elevated levels in patients with extensive disease [34].

Neuron-specific enolase (NSE) is a specific marker for neurons in the central and peripheral nervous system [31]. NSE has been found to be highly localized in the neuroendocrine, peptide secreting cells of the gut, pancreas, skin and lung. Levels of NSE in continuous cultures of SCLC were much higher than those observed in non-SCLC cells (Table 1). In a study of serum NSE levels in a large number of patients with SCLC, serum NSE levels demonstrated an excellent correlation with extent of disease. While elevated serum NSE was observed in 69% of all patients ($N = 94$), 100% of patients with 3 or more metastatic sites had an elevated serum NSE. In addition, in sequential studies of 23 patients, an excellent correlation between serum NSE levels and the observed clinical response to therapy was observed [33].

These *in vitro* studies of biologic markers in continuous cell lines of SCLC and non-SCLC lung cancer clearly demonstrate that DDC, CK-BB, bombesin and NSE determinations can distinguish cells of SCLC origin from those of other histologic types of lung cancer. As some of these 'markers' are released into the serum, their measurement in patients with SCLC may be useful in the staging and treatment of these patients. Further studies are required to demonstrate the specificity of these markers in patients with a variety of cancers, including other forms of lung cancer. The biologic function of these substances in SCLC remains undetermined, but preliminary studies with bombesin suggests that it may function as a growth-promoting factor for SCLC [36].

4. *IN VITRO* CLONING OF CLINICAL SPECIMENS OF SMALL CELL LUNG CANCER

At the present time the identification of new antineoplastic agents with potential value in the clinical management of patients with tumors is for the most part selected on the basis of *in vivo* results using a panel of animal tumors [37]. While such assays are essential for understanding the pharmacology and pharmakinetics of the agent, these *in vivo* tests of antineoplastic activity are both time-consuming and often unreliable. Recently considerable interest has been directed in the use of *in vitro* assay systems both for the selection of specific chemotherapy for individual patients, and for the screening of new agents in a Phase I–II situation. It is hoped that an *in vitro* assay using human tumors may be more reliable and less time-consuming than the present method for drug selection for clinical trials. Although many tests have been described for *in vitro* drug selection, including measurement of cell viability (vital dye exclusion, ^{51}Cr release), measurements of inhibition of cellular metabolism, and tests utilizing incorporation of radioactive precursors, the majority of these assays have not proved useful in chemotherapy selection or prediction. In many of these tests, the measurements are on the total cell population rather than the malignant cells and this may account for their limited use [38–40].

Kinetic data in human tumors and data generated from studies of bone marrow cells have suggested that within a given tumor cell population only a small fraction of the cells are responsible for the continual growth of the tumor – the so-called 'stem cells' or 'progenitor cells'. If this hypothesis is correct, then to be of use in chemotherapy selection an *in vitro* assay should selectively determine the effects of cytotoxic agents on this population alone, and not the admixed normal cells or other nonproliferating tumor cells.

In 1977, Drs Hamburger and Salmon first published on their success on the *in vitro* cloning in a semi-solid medium of 'stem' cells from a variety of human tumors, most notably multiple myeloma and ovarian carcinoma [41, 42]. Cytologic examination of histochemical and functional assays confirmed the tumor cell origin of the cells [42]. Subsequently the same authors and co-workers demonstrated that this *in vitro* clonogenic assay ('human tumor stem cell assay') could be used to quantitate the differential sensitivity of human tumors (ovarian and multiple myeloma) to anticancer agents [42, 43].

Since that time there have been many reports on the *in vitro* agarose cloning of a wide range of human tumors, including lung cancer [44–54]. Using a modification of the assay system originally described by Hamburger and Salmon, we have developed an *in vitro* culture system to assay for clonogenic ('?stem') cells in clinical specimens of small cell lung cancer. The detailed method for this assay has been previously described. Briefly, after clarification, a single cell suspension of the clinical specimen is plated in 0.3% agarose in culture medium over a base layer of 0.5% agarose which has hardened [49]. Specimens are incubated in a well-humidified atmosphere and colonies (cell aggregates of more than 50 cells) are usually observed 14–21 days after plating.

Our overall data for *in vitro* agarose cloning of clinical specimens obtained from patients with small cell lung cancer are shown in Table 2. Three hundred eighteen specimens were evaluated for cloning: 80 specimens contained histocytopathologically identifiable SCLC tumor cells in the biopsy or aspirate specimens, and the remainder were negative for tumor cells. *In*

Table 2. *In vitro* agarose colony formation of clinical specimens of small cell lung cancer.

| Source | No. | SCLC colony formation | |
		SCLC negative	SCLC positive
Bone marrow	261	0/226	34/35 (97%)
Pleural effusion	28	0/8	16/20 (76%)
Lymph node	20	0/0	15/20 (75%)
Liver	8	0/4	3/4 (75%)
Brain	1	0/0	1/1 (100%)
Total	318	0/238	69/80 (86%)

vitro SCLC agarose cloning was observed in 86% of the specimens containing tumor cells. The number of colonies ranges from 3–350 per 10^5 viable mononuclear cells plated with a median number of colonies per plate of 23. Specimens were cultured from a variety of metastatic sites including bone marrow, pleural effusions, lymph nodes, liver (specimens obtained under direct vision at periteoneoscopy) and a single surgically resected brain metastases. There was no significant difference in the ability to culture SCLC colonies from these various sites, and no difference in the colony forming efficiency in specimens obtained from newly diagnosed patients or previously untreated patients. Because SCLC is rarely surgically resected, no primary biopsy specimens were cultured in agarose. Although several attempts were made to culture SCLC colonies from bronchial washings, because of frequent contamination, no success was achieved and further attempts were not made. However, others have reported that bronchial washings can be used to clone lung cancer tumor cells[55].

The SCLC tumor cell origin and the 'stem cell' nature of cultured colonies were confirmed by cytological examination of multiple colonies from positive plates, by DNA content analysis, by flow cytometry of pooled agarose colonies, by electron microscopy examination of colonies, by inoculat-

Table 3. Demonstration of tumor cell origin and stem cell nature of agarose colonies[a].

Test	No. positive
SCLC cytology	69/69
Nude mouse tumor	10/12
Aneuploid DNA	10/10
Neurosecretory granules	2/2
Continuous growth	20/220

[a] Small cell lung cancer specimens.

ing colonies into athymic nude mice, and by attempting to subculture individual colonies in liquid culture [49, 56, 57] (Table 3). Cytology examination and electron microscopy examination always revealed cells with the typical morphological characteristics of SCLC. DNA content analysis in each instance revealed a single population of cells with a DNA content, usually aneuploid, identical to that of the tumor cells in the original clinical specimen confirming that only growth of tumor cells was occurring in the assay and that culture of cells in the agarose did not alter their DNA content.

When pooled colonies were inoculated intracranially into athymic nude mice, SCLC tumor formation was observed in 80% of the 12 specimens inoculated. The number of colonies inoculated into each mouse ranged from 2–20 (approximately 10^2–10^3 tumor cells). Typical signs of intracranial tumor appeared after latent periods ranging from 9 to 18 weeks. Unless mice were sacrificed immediately after the onset of symptoms, death occurred very rapidly. In 5/8 attempts, continuous cell lines of SCLC, with all the typical biological and biochemical characteristics of other cell lines of SCLC, were established in liquid culture from these nude mice tumors.

Although numerous attempts were made, successful culture of individual colonies to mass culture as continuous cell lines was not successful. Only 20 colonies (all from the same patient) were successfully propagated in culture when transferred from agarose to liquid culture. These data are in sharp contrast to subculturing individual colonies from cloned established cell lines, when approximately 75% of all individually picked colonies could be grown to mass culture [57]. The reasons for the failure to grow individual colonies after tansfer to liquid culture are unclear but most likely are related to growth factors and the need for other supporting cells for the initial growth of tumor cells [58].

Culture of SCLC colonies in specimens cytologically and histologically negative for SCLC tumor cells was not observed. These data are in contrast to those reported by others [59, 60]. Although tumor cell colony formation was observed in four specimens negative for tumor cells by routine pathological tests, a cytospin preparation of the specimen after processing for culture, and before a single cell suspension was obtained, always revealed the presence of tumor cells in specimens when resultant tumor cell colony was observed. Typical bone marrow stem cell colony was observed in several specimens cytologically negative for SCLC tumor cells. These colonies were morphologically distinct from SCLC colonies forming looser aggregates, and cytological examination of these colonies did not reveal any of the features of SCLC cells. These data would suggest that the clonogenic assay is not a useful additional screen of clinical specimens for the presence of tumor cells. There is no improved yield when a cytospin preparation is

Table 4. In vitro agarose cloning of clinical specimens of small cell lung cancer.

No. of specimens	318
No. of SCLC positive	80
No. of SCLC colony growth	69 (86%)
No. of colonies/10^5 cells	3–350
Mean No. of colonies	64
Median No. of colonies	23
No. of suitable for *in vitro* drug testing	18/80 (22%)

examined in addition to routine pathological procedures. In addition, because of the slow growth rate of cells in agarose, colony formation and confirmation of the nature of the colonies are usually not available for three weeks from the time the specimens are received. The only value of the clonogenic assay as a screening tool for tumor cells would be in examining bone marrow which has been collected for future transplantation. Clearly, in this instance all techniques should be used to confirm that tumor cells are absent from the stored marrow, prior to reinfusion.

Although *in vitro* agarose cloning of SCLC tumor cells can be achieved in 86% of specimens containing tumor cells, because of the poor colony forming efficiency, and because most specimens contain only a small number of cells (usually less than 10×10^6 total cells of which the majority are nonmalignant), *in vitro* drug sensitivity studies were successfully obtained in only 18 specimens. This represents 23% of all SCLC positive specimens and only 7% of all the specimens processed for cloning (Table 4). For the *in vitro* drug sensitivity assay to be considered successful, control plates contained at least 30 colonies, and at least one drug was tested in triplicate over a three-log concentration range. Using drugs with known clinical activity in SCLC, the clonogenic assay accurately predicted *in vivo* resistance in 100% of cases and *in vivo* sensitivity in 75% of cases, data very similar to that reported for other human tumors [42, 43, 54]. However, it must be considered that many patients received combination chemotherapy making evaluation of *in vitro* assays with single agents 'difficult' to assess. In addition, in relapsed patients, although a mean of 4.5 drugs was tested, the clonogenic assay did not aid in their therapeutic management. This is similar to data reported by Salmon *et al.*, who found that in 'resistant' tumors the success rate in identifying an active drug *in vitro* is proportional to the number of drugs tested [61]. In their study, when eight drugs could be tested, at least one active agent could be identified in 80% of cases.

If the *in vitro* clonogenic assay is to achieve widespread use in the management of patients with SCLC, growth conditions must be identified which will greatly improve the cloning of these tumor cells thereby permitting *in vitro* drug testing on a greater number of specimens. In addition, if we are to be able to test eight or more drugs in each assay, we must encourage physicians to make available sufficient material to perform these assays. An alternate approach would be to culture the cells in liquid culture for a period of time to increase the number of tumor cells available for *in vitro* drug testing.

With this approach we tested a number of continuous cell lines of SCLC for their *in vitro* sensitivity to cytotoxic agents and correlated the *in vitro* responses of these cell lines with the previously observed clinical response with the same drugs. Although in culture for prolonged periods (ranging from 4–60 months), the cell lines accurately predicted the *in vivo* responses for resistance in 100% of cases and sensitivity in 92% of tests. The cell lines tested included lines established from both newly diagnosed and previously treated patients. Thus, these data suggest that culture of SCLC tumor cells does not alter their chemosensitivity and that they may be of value in the screening of new cytotoxic agents with potential clinical activity in SCLC [62, 63]. Already, we have shown that these human cell lines are an excellent *in vitro* model for studies of drug metabolism and for understanding and evaluating mechanisms of drug sensitivity and resistance [64]. The data also suggest that fresh specimens may be initially cultured and then tested for *in vitro* sensitivity when sufficient tumor cells are available and when the cloning efficiency has increased [12].

5. SERUM-FREE CHEMICALLY DEFINED MEDIUM FOR THE GROWTH OF ESTABLISHED CELL LINES AND CLINICAL SPECIMENS OF SMALL CELL LUNG CANCER

The use of serum-supplemented medium for the growth of clinical specimens of human tumors has many disadvantages. A major problem is that growth of cells with serum is nonselective and thus overgrowth of normal nonmalignant stromal cells to the exclusion of the malignant cells is not uncommon. Serum contains both stimulatory and inhibitory substances such that growth responses may be poor and erratic. In addition, serum contains a variety of unknown compounds which may bind or inactivate exogenous factors making their growth promoting activity inevaluable. Serum proteins may bind or inactivate added cytotoxic agents giving false *in vitro* sensitivity results. Finally, with serum the growth-promoting properties may vary from batch to batch, and contamination with mycoplasma may occur.

Following the initial work of Sato *et al.*, and others [65–67], we attempted to define a serum-free, chemically supplemented medium which

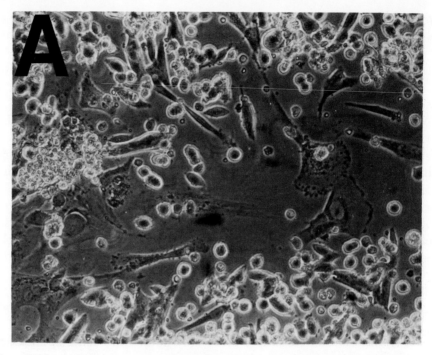

Figure 2. Morphological appearance of a clinical specimen of small cell lung cancer cultured in serum-supplemented medium (A) and serum-free chemically defined HITES medium. In serum-suplemented medium growth of both nonmalignant adherent stromal cells in addition to the floating SCLC cells is observed. In contrast (B) in the selective HITES medium only growth and proliferation of SCLC tumor cells is observed to the exclusion of all other cells no matter what their initial concentration.
(Reproduced with permission of Proc Natl Acad Sci 78:3185-3189, 1981 [12].)

would support the continual replication of SCLC cell lines *in vitro*. Although a large number of growth factors were tested, the combination of hydrocortisone, insulin, transferrin, estradiol and selenium, when added to RPMI 1640 medium (HITES medium) without serum, was demonstrated to support the growth of cell lines of SCLC at a rate similar to that observed in serum-supplemented medium [68].

The ability of this medium to support the growth of fresh clinical specimens was tested in a similar manner [12, 36]. Specimens, obtained from a variety of metastatic sites, were cultured in HITES medium and simultaneously in serum-supplemented medium (SSM, RPMI 1640 medium supplemented with 10% heat inactivated fetal bovine serum). The overall results for 41 specimens showed that while growth in SSM was observed in only 45% of the specimens, tumor cell proliferation was observed in the HITES medium in 70% of the same specimens. In HITES medium, only

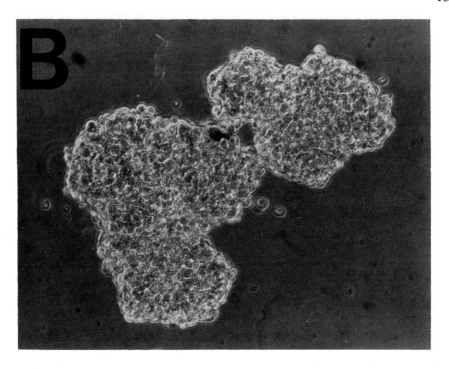

growth of the tumor cells was observed such that 7–14 days after plating, death of all normal cells had occurred and a pure population of rapidly dividing tumor cells was obtained. In contrast in SSM, proliferation of both tumor cells and nonmalignant stromal cells was observed. Growth of tumor cells in HITES medium was obtained in specimens obtained from newly diagnosed and previously treated patients and in specimens obtained from a variety of metastatic sites (Figure 2).

The selectivity of the HITES medium for the growth of fresh SCLC tumor specimens was tested by culturing bone marrow specimens cytologically negative for tumor cells and by culturing a wide variety of other human tumors, including non-SCLC lung cancers in the HITES medium. For cytologically negative specimens ($N = 100$), no growth of cells was observed in the HITES medium. By seven days, all cells were dead. In only 2 of 20 non-SCLC human tumor specimens was growth observed. A single adenocarcinoma of the lung specimens demonstrated growth for four weeks but died at this time. A mucoepidermoid cell carcinoma of the lung also grew in HITES medium and has been established as a continuous cell line in this medium.

The nature of the cells growing in the HITES medium was confirmed by cytology examination, by DNA content analysis, by flow cytometry, by nude mouse tumorigenicity, and by biochemical testing for *in vitro* SCLC markers. All of these studies confirmed that the cells growing in the HITES medium were malignant SCLC tumor cells. No differences in cytology or biochemical characteristics were observed in specimens cultured in both serum-supplemented medium and in HITES medium.

Although initial growth in HITES medium was rapid, in most instances, after 5–6 passages, cell growth rate slowed and occasionally ceased. The addition of 10% fetal bovine serum at this time supported the continual replication of the tumor cells. In approximately 20% of specimens, continual replication of tumor cells was observed in the HITES medium. These cell lines have now been maintained for periods ranging from six months to two years. It is unclear why some specimens can be maintained in serum-free medium indefinitely, while others cannot. Recently we have evaluated these cell lines to determine if they produce 'autocrine' growth-promoting factors. Preliminary evidence suggests that this is so (vide infra).

Because of the difficulty in maintaining all clinical specimens in a serum-free, chemically defined medium, we have recently evaluated a wide range of other factors which are known to be produced by SCLC including AVP and bombesin. Studies using cell lines of SCLC have demonstrated that both these hormones can stimulate the growth of SCLC *in vitro*, and when combined with HITES medium 1% BSA, ethanolamine and phosphoethanolamine (SCLC-2 medium [36]), growth of the cell lines is seen at a rate equal to or greater than that observed in serum-supplemented medium. Further studies are required to determine if this medium can improve the growth of fresh specimens.

6. 'AUTOCRINE STIMULATION' AND SMALL CELL LUNG CANCER

Considerable evidence exists that a variety of tumor cells produce factors which stimulate their own growth and proliferation ('autocrine stimulation') [69]. While the growth of nonmalignant cells requires the presence of a variety of exogenous polypeptides and hormones, the growth requirements of malignant cells are less stringent. The reasons postulated for this include the concept of autostimulation.

Recent data by Todaro *et al.* [70] would suggest that for some tumor cells such a growth-promoting mechanism exists. In their initial studies they clearly demonstrated that murine 3T3 cells transformed by Moloney Sarcoma virus could produce polypeptide 'transforming growth factors' (TGFs) or 'sarcoma growth factors'. This SGF is a potent mitogen, causes overgrowth and morphologic transformation of normal fibroblasts, and stimulates agarose colony formation of cells that under normal circumstances will not multiply in agarose [70]. Further studies using a variety of cell lines have demonstrated their ability to produce TGF [71].

More recently evidence has been produced to suggest that both SCLC and non-SCLC lung cancer cell lines produce TGF's [72]. In our initial experience in growing SCLC tumor cells from clinical specimens, the addition of 'conditioned medium' from an established cell line of SCLC greatly improved our ability to establish new cell lines of SCLC [8, 57]. In a recent report by Sherwin *et al.* [72], studies on 17 cell lines of lung cancer, including eight cell lines of SCLC, clearly demonstrated that the majority of these cell lines produced diffusible TGFs. In their assay system these factors could stimulate the *in vitro* agarose cloning of normal rat kidney fibroblast cells. Although there appeared to be a correlation between the production of soft agar growth factors and the absence of receptors on the cell surface for epidermal growth factor, the production of TGFs was a general property of lung cancer cells *in vitro* and independent of EGF receptors.

Recently we have further evaluated the autocrine phenomenon in cell lines of SCLC which have been permanently established in a serum-free, chemically defined medium (HITES medium). The ability of these cells to survive continually in the absence of serum-supplementation would suggest that these cells produce autostimulating factors. Although both clinical specimens and cell lines of SCLC could be cultured in liquid medium in serum-free HITES medium, *in vitro* agarose colony formation in HITES medium either did not occur or did so at a very low efficiency ($<10\%$ of that observed in serum-supplemented medium). Using conditioned medium from an established cell line in HITES (NCI N592), we observed that this conditioned medium (592 GF) promoted colony formation in serum-free HITES of itself at an efficiency equal to that observed in serum-supplemented medium. The 592 GF from this cell line promoted colony formation in agarose in serum-free medium with as little as 1.0% CM and promoted cloning of other cell lines of SCLC, but not of normal bone marrow or normal rat kidney fibroblasts [36]. The addition of this serum-free 592 CM to serum-supplemented medium also stimulated or increased colony formation, suggesting that the growth factors present in the conditioned medium are either absent or present in minute quantities in fetal bovine serum.

These data confirm that at least some cell lines of SCLC are capable of producing growth-promoting factors which are both autocrine and promote growth of other tumor cells. Whether the factors produced by these lung cancer cell lines are similar to SGF produced by other cells and whether the factors responsible for the clonal growth in serum-free medium of SCLC are the same factors are currently unknown. It is possible that these cells produce a variety of growth factors which can be assayed for in many different ways. The identification and characterization of such growth factors would greatly improve our ability to culture tumor cells. The characterization of receptors of such factors and the development of monoclonal antibodies to such receptors may offer a new approach to controlling tumor cell growth and proliferation [73].

7. CYTOGENETIC ANALYSIS OF SMALL CELL LUNG CANCER

With few exceptions cytogenetic analysis of solid tumor specimens has not been performed in a detailed fashion. The major difficulty has been that these tumors have few metaphases for study. However, DNA content analysis of human tumors can be easily performed using flow cytometry cells. A number of studies have reported on DNA content of SCLC tumor cells [74–76]. In approximately 65–75% of patients, in whom tumor cells were identified pathologically in the specimens, an aneuploid population of cells was identified in the sample with a DNA content ranging from 1.1 to 2.3 times diploid. In 10–20% of specimens, more than one aneuploid population of cells was identified suggesting that tumor cells with considerable heterogeneity may exist in these patients. Of interest, DNA content analysis of fresh specimens may serve as a useful means for monitoring tumor cell proliferation when clinical specimens are plated in culture [76]. We have recently demonstrated that agarose colonies of SCLC do not change their DNA content after culture [56] and that cell lines of SCLC, for the most part, do not change their total DNA content with passage. These data suggest that frequent measurement of DNA content may be useful for screening of cross-contamination of cell lines in tissue culture laboratories.

Recently, using established cell lines of SCLC, we have demonstrated a specific cytogenetic abnormality associated with this tumor. In these cell lines, although frequent abnormalities of other chromosomes were present in some cell lines, all cell lines had a deletion of all or a portion of the short arm of chromosome 3 [77–79]. Shortest region of overlap analysis showed that the common region deleted was del (3) [14–23], often called an interstitial deletion. The abnormality was found in cell lines from males and females, from treated and untreated patients, and in lines established from a variety of metastatic sites. The abnormality was not identified in autologous B lymphoblastoid cell lines or in cell lines of other forms of lung cancer.

Using the selective medium (HITES) for growth of SCLC, we have evaluated fresh specimens, after 2–3 days culture, when rapid proliferation of only tumor cells is observed in this medium, for the presence of this cytogenetic abnormality. The 3p abnormality was identified in all fresh specimens examined confirming that its presence is not an artifact of culture, but rather a specific defect associated with SCLC. Whether the 3p abnormality is directly related to the malignant behavior of SCLC, or only associated with it, remains to be determined. Further studies are required to determine if the part of chromosome 3 is lost or translocated to another chromosome in SCLC.

8. NUDE MOUSE TUMORIGENICITY OF CLINICAL SPECIMENS AND CELL LINES OF SCLC

Since its original description, the nude athymic mouse has served as a useful means for evaluating the tumorigenicity of both fresh specimens and cell lines, and for studying the effects of chemotherapeutic agents on tumors established in nude mice [80, 81]. Both clinical specimens and established cell lines of SCLC readily form tumors when inoculated subcutaneously (SC) in these animals. Once established as a tumor in mice, these specimens can be readily heterotransplanted from one mouse to another with a high 'take' rate and can also be established as continuous cell lines in cultures [82–85]. These cell lines retain all the typical characteristics of SCLC grown directly from patient specimens.

Recently we, and others, have demonstrated that SCLC will form tumors in almost 100% of cases when inoculated intracranially (IC) into athymic nude mice [83, 85]. In addition, tumor formation is observed IC with 100–1000-fold less cells than that required to induce tumor formation SC [85]. This observation has permitted the *in vivo* evaluation of the 'stem cell' nature of agarose colonies cultured directly from patient specimens. In the majority of cases tested, tumors were formed from agarose colonies, confirming the nature of the colonies. Continuous cell lines could be established from these IC tumors in 50% of cases attempted. Thus the nude mouse serves as a useful mechanism for both the establishment of cell lines, and for the characterization of cells cultured directly from clinical specimens.

Several reports have evaluated the response of nude mouse heterotransplants to cytotoxic therapy and compared results to that observed clinically in the patients from whom the specimens were obtained [86]. Although only a small number of correlations could be made, results in the nude mouse were very similar to those observed in patients treated with the same agents. These data suggest that nude mouse heterotransplants may be useful for evaluating new drugs with potential activity in the treatment of SCLC. Whether nude mouse sensitivity data can be used to treat patients on an individual basis is unlikely as considerable time may elapse between the inoculation of specimens into the mice and the development of the tumor. In many instances, the patients have died before successful tumor formation is observed.

9. TRANSFORMATION OF SMALL CELL LUNG CANCER TO LARGE CELL CARCINOMA

Clinical studies of patients with SCLC have demonstrated that at diagnosis approximately 6% will be a mixed small cell/large cell histology [16, 17]. Patients with the mixed histology have a poorer response rate and shorter median survival than those with 'pure' SCLC [87]. In addition, autopsy studies of patients with SCLC have revealed that up to 35% of patients will have a mixed histology. Whether this 'change' in histology is related to chemotherapy or is due to the emergence of a second tumor is unclear. This 'change' may also explain why patients with SCLC who relapse from primary therapy are now usually less responsive to further chemotherapy and radiation therapy [2].

In a small number of permanently established cell lines we, and others [11, 88] have observed a change in morphological appearance of cells from a typical SCLC appearance to a large cell morphology. This 'transformation' is associated with an increase in growth rate and cloning efficiency and also a loss of typical APUD characteristics including L-dopa decarboxylase and neurosecretory granules.

The clinical significance of this change can be demonstrated by the observation that when this *in vitro* transformation occurs, the transformed cells demonstrate a marked resistance to radiation in contrast to 'classic' SCLC cells [88, 89]. Whether this resistance is directly related to the loss of APUD properties, or merely associated with the changes remains to be determined. The increased resistance to radiation with changing histology may explain the poor responses to cytotoxic therapy observed in patients with relapse from primary therapy.

10. SUMMARY

Although there are four major histologic types of lung cancer, only SCLC remains curable with combination cytotoxic therapy. Considerable advances in our understanding of the biology of this tumor have occurred through our ability to establish continuous cell lines of SCLC. With these cell lines we have confirmed the APUD properties of SCLC including the presence of neurosecretory granules and high levels of the key APUD enzyme L-dopa decarboxylase. The characterization of these lines has identified markers not previously associated with SCLC, including creatine-kinase BB, neuron-specific enolase, and bombesin. Although the functional role of these 'markers' has not yet been determined, data suggest that serum measurements of these markers may prove useful in both the staging and management of patients with SCLC.

Cell lines of SCLC have also permitted the characterization of specific growth requirements of this tumor such that now cell lines of SCLC can be readily established in a serum-free, chemically defined medium. Cells cultured in this HITES medium retain all the typical *in vitro* characteristics of SCLC. Further studies with other growth factors, using this defined HITES medium, may help identify factors with both growth-promoting and inhibitory properties for SCLC. Modulation of these factors *in vivo* may prove useful in controlling the growth of SCLC.

Although a large fraction of clinical specimens and cell lines of SCLC will have abnormal DNA contents as measured by flow cytometry and may serve as an *in vitro* marker for growth, more detailed studies of chromosomes in both cell lines and clinical specimens have demonstrated a specific cytogenetic abnormality in SCLC, a deletion involving chromosome 3. If confirmed by other investigators, then cytogenetic analysis of human lung cancer specimens may have an important role in the management of these patients.

We, and others, have reported on the *in vitro* agarose cloning of clinical specimens of SCLC. Although the nature of these colonies has been confirmed by biologic studies, two factors, notably the small volume of tumor specimen obtained and chiefly the poor colony-forming efficiency of these tumor cells, have prevented the widespread application of the clonogenic assay for *in vitro* chemotherapy selection for individual patients. Clearly before this assay can achieve routine use in oncology, these problems must be overcome. As different bacteria have different growth requirements, it must also be assumed that tumors of different histologic types must also have different growth requirements. For the cloning efficiency of tumors to be improved, such that successful *in vitro* drug testing can be performed on the majority of specimens, *in vitro* studies with tumors of different histology must be performed such that optimal growth requirements for each type can be identified.

Finally, with cell lines of SCLC we have developed monoclonal antibodies to SCLC (see Chapter 2). The development of monoclonal antibodies specific to SCLC may have potential benefit in both the diagnosis and treatment of patients with this disease. Their use offers an alternative approach in the management of these patients.

REFERENCES

1. Cancer statistics 1980: CA – A Cancer Journal for Clinicians 31:13–28, 1981.
2. Minna JD, Higgins GA, Glatsten EJ: Cancer of the lung. In: Principles and Practice of Oncology. DeVita VT *et al.* (eds). Philadelphia: JB Lippincott, 1981, pp. 396–474.

3. Straus MJ: The growth characteristics of lung cancer and its application to treatment design. Serum Oncol 1:167–174, 1974.
4. Muggia FM, Krezoski SK, Hansen HH: Cell kinetic studies in patients with small cell lung cancer. Cancer 34:1683–1690, 1974.
5. Matthews MJ, Kanhouwa S, Pickren J, Robinette, D: Frequency of residual and metastatic tumor in patients undergoing curative surgical resection for lung cancer. Cancer Chemother Rep 4:63–67, 1973.
6. Pearse AGE: The cytochemistry and ultrastructure of polypeptide hormone producing cells of the APUD series and the embryologic, physiologic and pathologic implications of the concept. J. Histochem Cytochem 17:303–313, 1969.
7. Bonikos DS, Bensch KG: Endocrine cells of bronchial and bronchiolar epithelium. Am J Med 63:765-711, 1977.
8. Gazdar AF, Carney DN, Russell, EK, et al.: Small cell carcinoma of the lung; establishment of continuous clonable cell lines having APUD properties. Cancer Res 40:3502–3507, 1980.
9. Petengill OS, Sorenson GD, Wurster-Hill DH, et al.: Isolation and growth characteristics of continuous cell lines from small-cell carcinoma of the lung. Cancer 45:906–918, 1980.
10. Pettengill OS, Sorenson GD: Tissue culture and *in vitro* characteristics of small cell lung cancer. In: Small Cell Lung Cancer. Greco FA, et al. (eds). New York: Grune & Stratton, 1981, pp 51–79.
11. Gazdar AF, Carney DN, Guccion JG, Baylin SB: Small cell carcinoma of the lung: cellular origin and relationship to other pulmonary tumors. In: Small Cell Lung Cancer. Greco FA, et al. (eds). New York: Grune & Stratton, 1981, pp 145–177.
12. Carney DN, Bunn PA Jr, Gazdar AF, Pagan JA, Minna JD: Selective growth of small cell carcinoma of the lung obtained from patient biopsies in serum-free hormone supplemented medium. Proc Natl Acad Sci USA 78:3185–3189, 1981.
13. Baylin SB, Abeloff MD, Goodwin G, et al.: Activities of L-dopa decarboxylase and diamine oxidase (histaminase) in lung cancers and decarboxylase as a marker for small (oat) cell cancer in culture. Cancer Res 40:1990-1994, 1980.
14. Baylin SB, Weisburger WR, Eggleston JC, et al.: Variable content of histaminase, L-dopa decarboxylase and calcitonin in small-cell carcinoma of the lung: biologic and clinical implications. N Eng J Med 299:105–110, 1978.
15. Gazdar AF, Zweig MH, Carney DN, et al.: Levels of creatine kinase and its isozyme in lung cancer tumors and cultures. Cancer Res 41:2773–2777, 1981.
16. Matthews MJ, Gazdar AF: Pathology of small cell carcinoma of the lung and its subtypes: a clinico-pathologic correlation. In: Lung Cancer. Livingston RB (ed). The Hague: Martinus Nijhoff Publishers, 1981, pp 283–386.
17. Abeloff MD, Eggleston JC, Mendelsohn G, Ettinger DS, Baylin SB: Changes in morphologic and biochemical characteristics of small cell carcinoma of the lung: a clinico-pathologic study. Am J Med 66:757–764, 1979.
18. Richardson RL, Greco FA, Oldham RK, Liddle GW: Tumor products and potential tumor markers in small cell lung cancer. Semin Oncol 5(3):253–262, 1978.
19. Hansen M, Hammer M, Hummer L: Diagnostic and therapeutic implications of ectopic hormone production in small cell carcinoma of the lung. Thorax 35:101–106, 1980.
20. Wallach S, Royston I, Wohl H, Newman DR, Deftos L: Plasma calcitonin as a marker of disease activity in patients with small cell carcinoma of the lung. J Clin Endocrinol and Metab 53:602–606, 1981.
21. Waalkes TP, Abeloff MA, Woo KB, Ettinger DS, Ruddon RW, Aldenderfer T: Carcinoembryonic antigen for monitoring patients with small cell carcinoma of the lung during treatment. Cancer Res 40:4420–4427, 1980.

22. North WG, Maurer H, Valtin H, O'Donnell JF: Human neurophysins as potential markers for small cell carcinoma of the lung: applications of specific radioimmunoassay. J Endocrinol Metab 51:892–896, 1980.

23. Gropp C, Havemann K, Scheurer A: Ectopic hormones in lung cancer patients at diagnosis and drug therapy. Cancer 46:347–354, 1980.

24. Hansen M, Hammer M, Hummer L: ACTH, ADH, and calcitonin concentrations as markers for response and relapse in small cell carcinoma of the lung. Cancer 46:2062–2067, 1980.

25. Woo KB, Waalkes P, Abeloff MA, Ettinger DS, McNitt KL, Gehrke CW: Multiple biologic markers in the monitoring of treatment for small cell carcinoma of the lung: the use of serial levels of plasma CEA and carbohydrates. Cancer 48:1633-1642, 1981

26. Hansen M: Clinical implications of ectopic hormone production in small cell carcinoma of the lung. Danish Med Bulletin 28:221–236, 1981.

27. Greco FA, Hainsworth J, Sismani A, Richardson RL, Hande KR, Oldham RK: Hormone production and paraneoplastic syndromes. In: Small Cell Lung Cancer. Greco FA, et al. (eds). New York: Grune & Stratton, 1981, pp 177–225.

28. Sorenson GD, Pettengill OS, Brink-Johnson T, et al.: Hormone production by cultures of small cell carcinoma of the lung. Cancer 47:1289–1296, 1981.

29. Gazdar AF, Zweig MH, Carney DN, et al.: Levels of creatine kinase and its isozyme in lung cancer tumors and cultures. Cancer Res 41:2773–2777, 1981.

30. Moody TW, Pert CB, Gazdar AF, Carney DN, Minna JD: High levels of intracellular bombesin characterize human small cell lung carcinoma. Science 214:1246–1248, 1981.

31. Marangos PJ, Gazdar AF, Carney DN: Neuron Specific enolase in human small cell carcinoma cultures. Cancer Let. 15:67–71, 1982.

32. Carney DN, Zweig MH, Minna JD, et al.: Creatine-kinase BB: a clinical marker for tumor burden in patients with small cell carcinoma of the lung. AFCR: 433A, 1981.

33. Carney DN, Marangos PJ, Ihde DC, Cohen MH, Minna JD, Gazdar AF: Neuron specific enolase: a marker for disease extent and response to therapy in patients with small cell lung cancer. Lancet 1:583–585, 1982.

34. Pert CB, Schumacher UK: Plasma bombesin concentration in patients with extensive small cell lung cancer. Lancet 1:509, 1981.

35. Wood SM, Wood JR, Ghatel MA, Lee YC, O'Shaughnessy D, Bloom SR: Bombesin, somatostatin and neurolensin-like immunoreactivity in bronchial carcinoma. J Endocrinol and Metab 53:1310–1312, 1981.

36. Minna JD, Carney DN, Oie H, Bunn PA, Gazdar AF: Growth of human small cell lung cancer in defined medium. In: Growth of Cells in Defined Medium, Vol. 9. Pardee A and Sato G (eds). New York: Cold Spring Harbor Press, 1982, pp. 627–639.

37. Venditti JM: Preclinical drug development: rationale and methods. Semin Oncol 4: 349–361, 1981.

38. Von Hoff DD, Weisenthal L: In vitro methods to predict for patient response to chemotherapy. Advances in Pharmacol and Chemother vii:133–156, 1980.

39. Hamburger AW: Uses of in vitro tests in predictive cancer chemotherapy. J Natl Cancer Inst 66:981–988, 1981.

40. Weisenthal L: In vitro assays in preclinical anlineoplastic drug screening. Semin Oncol 4:362–377, 1981.

41. Hamburger AW, Salmon SE: Primary bioassay of human tumor stem cells. Science 197:461–463, 1977.

42. Hamburger AW, Salmon SE: Primary bioassay of human myeloma stem cells. J Clin Invest 60:846–854, 1977.

43. Salmon SE, Hamburger AW, Soehnlen B, Durie BGM, Alberts DS, Moon TE: Quantitation

of differential sensitivity of human tumor stem cells to anticancer drugs. N Engl J Med 298:1321–1327, 1978.

44. Alberts DS, Chen HSG, Soehnlen B, Salmon SE, Surwitt EA, Young L, Moon TE: *In vitro* clonogenic assay for predicting response of ovarian cancer to chemotherapy. Lancet 2: 340–342, 1980.

45. Courtenay VD, Selby PJ, Smith IE, Mills J, Peckhan MJ: Growth of human tumor cell colonies from biopsies using the two soft-agar techniques. Brit J Cancer 38:77–82, 1978.

46. Hamburger AW, Salmon SE, Kim MB, Trent JM, Soehnlen BJ, Alberts DC, Schmidt HJ: Direct cloning of human ovarian carcinoma cells in agar. Cancer Res 38:3438–3444, 1978.

47. Kinball PM, Brattain MG, Pitts AM: A soft-agar procedure measuring growth of human colonic carcinoma. Br J Cancer 37:1015–1019.

48. Buick RN, Stanistic TH, Fry SE, Salmon SE, Trent JM, Krasovic P: Development of an agar-methyl cellulose clonogenic assay for cells in transitional cell carcinoma of the bladder. Cancer Res 39:5051–5056, 1979.

49. Carney DN, Gazdar AF, Minna JD: Positive correlation between histologic tumor involvement and generation of tumor cell colonies in agarose in specimens taken directly from patients with small cell carcinoma of the lung. Cancer Res 40:1820–1823, 1980.

50. Ozols RF, Wilson IKV, Grotzinger KR, Young RC: Cloning of human ovarian cells in soft agar from malignant effusions and peritoneal washings. Cancer Res 40:2743–2747, 1980.

51. Rosenblum MD, Vasquez DA, Hoshine T, Wilson CB: Development of a clonogenic cell assay for human brain tumors. Cancer 41:2305–2314, 1978.

52. Von Hoff DD, Casper J, Bradley E, Trent JM, Hodach A, Reichert C, Makuch R, Altman A: Direct cloning of human neuroblastoma cells in soft agar culture. Cancer Res 40: 3591–3597, 1980.

53. Pavelic ZP, Slocum HK, Rustum YM, Creaven PJ, Nowak NJ, Karakousis C, Takita H, Mittelman A: Growth of cell colonies in soft agar from biopsies of different human solid tumors. Cancer Res 40:4151–4158, 1980.

54. Von Hoff DD, Casper J, Bradley E, *et al.*: Association between human tumor colony-forming assay results and response of an individual patient's tumor to chemotherapy. Am J Med 70:1027–1032, 1981.

55. Von Hoff DD, Weisenthal LW, Ihde DC, *et al.*: Growth of lung cancer colonies from bronchoscopy washings. Cancer, 1981.

56. Carney DN, Gazdar AF, Bunn PA Jr, Guccion JG: Demonstration of the stem cell nature of clonogenic tumor cells from lung cancer patients. Stem Cells 1:149–164, 1981.

57. Carney DN, Gazdar AF, Bunn PA Jr, Minna JD: *In vitro* cloning of small cell carcinoma of the lung. In: Small Cell Lung Cancer Greco FA (eds). New York: Grune & Stratton, 1981, pp 74–94.

58. Buick RN, Fry SE, Salmon SE: Effect of host cell interactions on clonogenic carcinoma cells in human malignant effusions. Brit J Cancer 41:695–704, 1980.

59. Pollard EB, Ferman T, Myers W, *et al.*: Utilization of a human tumor cloning system to monitor for marrow involvement with small cell carcinoma of the lung. Cancer Res 41:1015–1020, 1981.

60. Callaghan SK, Von Hoff DD: Growth of oat cell carcinoma of the lung in human tumor cloning assay. Presented at Third Conference of Human Tumor Cloning, Arizona. Abstract 17, 1982.

61. Dana D, Meyskens FL, Franks DH, *et al.*: *In vitro* chemosensitivity of human melanoma tumor stem cells in soft agar and *in vitro/in vivo* correlations. Proc ASCO/AACR 22:C-749, 1981.

62. Salmon S, Alberts A, Mayskens F, Durei B, Jones S, Soehnlen B, Young L: A new concept

in vitro phase II trial with the human tumor stem cell assay. Proc AACR/ASCO 20:C-41, 1980.

63. Carney DN, Gazdar AF, Minna JD: *In vitro* chemosensitivity of clinical specimens and cell lines of small cell lung cancer. Proc AACR/ASCO, 1982 (in press).

64. Curt GA, Jolivet J, Carney DN, Bailey B, Clendennin N, Cowan K, Chaber BA: Methotrexate resistance in human small cell lung cancer cells. Proc AACR/ASCO, 1982 (in press).

65. Hayashi I, Sato G: Replacement of serum by hormones permits the growth of cells in a defined medium. Nature 259:132-134, 1976.

66. Ham RG, McKeehan WL: In: Methods in Eneymology, Vol 43. Jacoby WB and Pastan IH (eds). New York: Academic Press, 1979, pp 44-93.

67. Barnes D, Sato G: Methods for growth of cultured cells in serum-free medium. Analytical Biochem 102:255-270, 1980.

68. Simms E, Gazdar AF, Abrams PG, Minna JD: Growth of human small cell (oat cell) carcinoma of the lung in serum-free growth factor-supplemented medium. Cancer Res 40:4356-4361, 1980.

69. Sporn MB, Todaro GJ: Autocrine secretion and malignant transformation of cells. N Eng J Med 303:878-880, 1980.

70. Todaro GJ, De Larco JE: Growth factors produced by sarcoma virus-transformed cells. Cancer Res 38:4147-4154, 1978.

71. Todaro GJ, Fryling C, De Larco JE: Transforming growth factors produced by certain human tumor cells: polypeptides that interact with epidermal growth factor receptors. Proc Natl Acad Sci 77:5258-5262, 1980.

72. Sherwin SA, Minna JD, Gazdar AF, Todaro GJ: Expression of epidermal and nerve growth factor receptors and soft agar growth factor production by human lung cancer cells. Cancer Res 41:3538-3542, 1981.

73. Trowbridge IS, Lopez F: Monoclonal antibody to transferrin receptor blocks transferrin binding and inhibits tumor cell growth *in vitro*. Proc Natl Acad Sci 79: 1175-1179, 1982.

74. Bunn PA, Jr Schlam M, Gazdar AF: Comparison of cytology and DNA content analysis in specimens from lung cancer patients. Proc AACR/ASCO 21:160, 1980.

75. Vindelov LL, Spang-Thomsen M, Engelholm SA, Christensen, IJ, Visfeldt J, Nissen NI: Clonal heterogeneity of small cell carcinoma of the lung demonstrated *in vivo* and *in vitro*. Presented at XIth ESGCP Meeting, Adthus, Denmark, 1981.

76. Bunn PA, Jr, Carney DN, Gazdar AF, Minna JD: Stability of DNA content in long-term cell lines of small cell lung cancer (personal communication).

77. Whang-Peng J, Kao-Shun CS, Lee EC, Bunn PA, Carney DN, Gazdar AF, Minna JD: A specific chromosome defect associated with human small cell lung cancer: deletion 3p (14-23). Science 215:181-183, 1982.

78. Whang-Peng JW, Bunn PA, Kao-Shun CS, Lee EC, Carney DN, Minna JD, Gazdar AF: A non-randomal chromosomal abnormality, del 3p (14-23) in human small cell lung cancer. Cancer Gen Cytogenet 6:119-134, 1982.

79. Whang-Peng J, Kao-Shun CS, Lee EC, Bunn PA, Carney DN, Gazdar AF, Portlock C, Minna JD: Human small cell lung cancer: deletion 3p (14-23) double minute chromosomes, and homogeneously staining regions in human small cell lung cancer. In: Gene Amplification, the Banbury report. New York: Cold Spring Harbor Lab Press, 1982, pp 107-114.

80. Shimosato Y, Kayema T, Tvagi K, *et al.*: Transplantation of human tumors into nude mice. J. Natl Cancer Inst 56:1251-1260, 1876.

81. Reid L, Shins M, Fogh J, Giovanelle B (eds). The Nude Mouse in Experimental and Clinical Research. New York: Academic Press, 1978, pp 313-351.

82. Pettengill OS, Curphey TJ, Cate CC, Flint CF, Maurer LH, Sorenson GD: Animal model

for small cell carcinoma of the lung; effect of immunosuppression and sex of mouse on tumor growth in athymic nude mice. Exp Cell Biol 48:279–297, 1980.

83. Chambers WF, Pettengill OS, Sorenson GD: Intercranial growth of pulmonary small cell carcinoma cells in nude athymic mice. Exp Cell Biol 49:90–97, 1981.

84. Sorenson GD, Pettengill OS, Cate CC: Studies on xenografts of small cell carcinoma of the lung. In: Small Cell Lung Cancer. Greco FA, et al. (eds). New York: Grune & Stratton, 1981, pp 95–122.

85. Gazdar AF, Carney DN, Sims HL, Simmons A: Heterotransplantation of small cell carcinoma of the lung into nude mice. 1. comparison of intracranial and subcutaneous routes. Int V Cancer 28:777–783, 1981.

86. Shorthouse AJ, Smyth JF, Steel GG, Ellison M, Mills J, Peckham MH: The human tumor xenograft – a valid model in experimental chemotherapy. Br J. Surg 67:715–722, 1980.

87. Radice PA, Matthers MJ, Ihde DC, et al.: The clinical behavior of mixed small cell/large cell bronchogenic carcinoma compared to 'pure' small cell subtypes. Cancer, 1982 (in press).

88. Goodwin G, Baylin SB: In vitro, marked differences in ultrastructure, biochemistry and response to X-irradiation separate the large cell variant of small cell lung carcinoma from classic small cell carcinoma. Proc AACR/ASCO 21:187, 1981.

89. Carney DN, Mitchell JB, Kinsella TJ: Development of radiation resistance associated with transformation of human small cell lung cancer to large cell variants. Proc AACR/ASCO 22:631, 1982.

2. Monoclonal Antibodies Against Human Lung Cancer: Potential Diagnostic and Therapeutic Use

FRANK CUTTITTA, STEVEN ROSEN, DESMOND N. CARNEY, ADI F. GAZDAR and JOHN D. MINNA

1. INTRODUCTION

Since the advent of Kohler and Milstein's somatic cell hybridization technique [1], a true renaissance in tumor cell biology has been achieved with the use of monoclonal antibodies. These molecular probes not only have potential diagnostic and therapeutic value but also allow for the dissection of cellular events which occur at the molecular level of neoplasms. In the past pentad several laboratories have attempted to develop monoclonal antibodies which would distinguish human tumor cells from their non-malignant (normal) counterparts. Such discriminatory reagents have been reported for neuroblastomas [2], gliomas [3], colon cancer [4–6], breast cancer [7], lymphomas [8], leukemias [9, 10] and malignant melanoma [11–14]. Recently, the hybridoma technique has been applied for the development of monoclonal antibodies to human lung cancer [15–18].

Pulmonary malignancies affect over 100,000 new patients each year and characteristically present as four major histological types: adenocarcinoma, large cell carcinoma, squamous carcinoma and small cell carcinoma [19–21]. These pleural neoplasm vary in their clinical behavior and assigned course of treatment. For example, patients who present with small cell lung cancer (SCLC) are usually beyond the bounds of surgical resection and are treated with chemotherapy with or without radiotherapy [19]. Non-small cel lung malignancies, being resistant to chemotherapy, are routinely treated with surgery or radiotherapy [19]. Though distinct morphological differences clearly discern 'classical' SCLC from non-SCLC tumors, atypical (variant) forms of neoplasms occur in about 6% of small cell carcinomas at presentation and can emulate other histological types of lung cancer [22]. Many biochemical and cytogenetic markers are now being used to better define SCLC and their variant morphological types [20, 23]. In an effort to establish new methods for early diagnosis, histological typing, staging and

Greco, FA (ed), Biology and Management of Lung Cancer. ISBN 0-89838-554-7.
© 1983, Martinus Nijhoff Publishers, Boston. Printed in The Netherlands.

rational selection of therapy for human lung cancer, our group has developed the technological means for the *in vitro* cultivation of SCLC [24–27]. The SCLC lines thus far produced have been verified to be of this specified tumor type by the following characteristics: the lines were started from patients with documented histology and a clinical course consistent with small cell carcinoma of the lung; all lines displayed human chromosomes and human isoenzymes; the lines induced tumors in nude mice and these heterotransplants showed a histology similar to that seen in the patient's tumor; the cells had the typical appearance of SCLC in suspension culture and formed colonies in soft agar; the lines expressed high specific activities of L-dopa decarboxylase, neuron-specific enolase and creatine-kinase BB isozyme; the cells exhibited neurosecretory granules and were shown to produce a variety of peptide hormones; and all lines were shown to have del 3p (14-23) chromosomal defect [24–31]. For a more detailed review on the characterization of SCLC cell lines, see Chapter 1 of this monograph.

Prompted by the availability of these well-characterized SCLC lines, we began to investigate the use of such lines as initial immunogens for the development of monoclonal antibodies. In several instances, autologous B-lymphoblastoid or skin fibroblast lines were concomitantly generated with their mate SCLC counterparts and were incorporated in our primary screening strategy to eliminate monoclonal antibodies directed against histocompatibility antigens. This chapter discusses the production, characterization and use of monoclonal antibodies that demonstrate specificity for several types of human lung cancer. We review the potential diagnostic and therapeutic values of such reagents and their usefulness as molecular probes for investigating the onconeogenic process.

2. ANTIBODIES TO HUMAN LUNG CANCER

We describe here a brief overview of our experimental approach and the screening strategy used for the derivation of monoclonal antibodies to human long cancer. For more detailed information concerning the hybridoma technology presented below, see Cuttitta *et al.* [15] and Minna *et al.* [16].

BALB/c mice or Sprague-Dawley, Fischer rats were hyperimmunized, over a 6-week period, with one or more viable SCLC lines (NCI-H69, NCI-H187 or NCI-H64) [24]. The resulting splenocytes were fused with one of three mouse myeloma cell lines (P3X63, P3-NS1-1-Ag4-1, X63-Ag8.653) [1, 32, 33] using the polyethylene glycol procedures of Galfre *et al.* [33]. Hybrids were selectively grown in 96-well microtiter plates using a modification of Kennett's formula [34]. Fourteen days following the fusion,

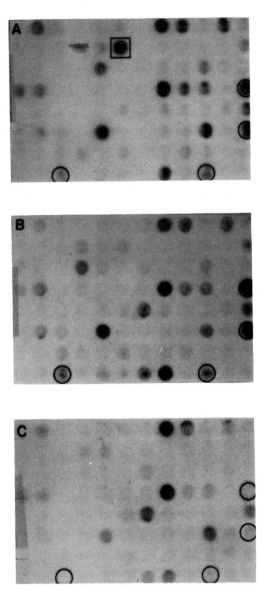

Figure 1. Example of the immunoradioautograph produced during the primary screening of hybridoma culture supernatants for anti-SCLC activity. Target cells were glutaraldehyde fixed to 96-well polyvinyl chloride plates: (A) SCLC line NCI-H69 (immunogen line); (B) SCLC line NCI-H128; (C) autologous B-lymphoblastoid line NCI-H128BL. Hybrid culture fluids were transferred to the respective target cell plates using a 96-well replicator device (thus maintaining spacial orientation of samples), attached mouse or rat immunoglobulins were detected employing a secondary antibody (rabbit antimouse/rat IgG-IgM) followed by ^{125}I-protein A. The deposition of radioactive tracer was evaluated by overnight autoradiography on Kodak XR-5 film using a Dupont lightning-plus intensifying screen.

individual culture supernatants were tested for anti-SCLC activity by immunoradioautography. This was accomplished using a solid phase system consisting of three target cell plates: the initial immunogen SCLC line NCI-H69, an additional SCLC line (NCI-H128) and its autologous B-lymphoblastoid line (NCI-H128BL). Hybridoma culture fluids were transferred to the appropriate target cell plates and bound monoclonal antibody was detected indirectly by the addition of a secondary antibody (rabbit antimouse or rat immunoglobulin, respectively) followed by ^{125}I-labeled staphylococcal protein-A. Figure 1 demonstrates the binding pattern observed in a routine test procedure. The circled wells represent those hybrids which were selective for SCLC and thus chosen for further studies. Employing this type of screening strategy, we were successful in eliminating those antibodies which recognized common antigens universally expressed on human cell lines (i.e., structural proteins, enzymes, etc.) and histocompatibility antigens (the boxed well in Figure 1 represents a possible HLA binding antibody). Positive SCLC reacting hybrids were stabilized by repeated 'minicloning' [35] and subsequently single cell cloned by 'limiting dilution' [16].

The numerical evaluation of our attempts to derive monoclonal antibodies with selective recognition for human SCLC is presented in Table 1. In 15 separate fusions, involving mouse × mouse or rat × mouse hybrids, 10,218 wells were tested using the previously described screening method; 1,102 of the wells (10.8%) gave positive reactions for at least one human target cell

Table 1. Numerical evaluation of the screening results generated during the testing of primary hybridoma culture fluids for selective monoclonal antibodies to human small cell lung cancer.

	Mouse[a]	Rat[b]	Total
Fusions	11	4	15
Total number wells seeded	8,448	1,770	10,218 (100.0)[c]
Wells with hybridoma cell growth	3,301	1,379	4,680 (45.8)
Wells showing any human cell reaction	699	403	1,102 (10.8)
Wells showing selective SCLC reaction[d]	115	73	188 (1.9)
Wells showing selective SCLC reaction following stabilization[e]	59	22	81 (0.8)

[a] Summary of mouse × mouse fusions using P3 × 63, 653 and NS1 parent myeloma cell lines.
[b] Summary of rat × mouse fusions using 653 and NS1 parent myeloma cell lines.
[c] Percentage of total wells tested.
[d] Positive radioautographic single for both SCLC lines NCI-69 and NCI-128 but negative on the NCI-128BL B-lymphoblastoid cell line.
[e] Maintained selective SCLC binding following the minicloning and single cell cloning process.

line; and only 188 wells (1.9%) showed selective reactivity for both SCLC lines. The technical difficulty in generating anti-SCLC producing hybridomas becomes even more evident when one considers that, of the 188 hybrids initially showing selective SCLC binding, less than 45% (81 wells) maintain their properties following single cell cloning. Thus, the overall efficiency in the derivation of anti-SCLC antibodies is 0.8%.

3. FURTHER CHARACTERIZATION OF MONOCLONAL ANTIBODIES SELECTIVE FOR HUMAN SCLC

Those hybridomas fulfilling the requirements of our initial screening restrictions were further assessed for their binding specificity. Our first approach in evaluating these reagents was to see if their selective binding was maintained when tested against different SCLC lines. Figure 2 represents the binding titration curve of a mouse monoclonal antibody (534F8) on three autologous pairs of cell lines. The antibody shows significant binding with the SCLC lines from three different patients (NCI-N390, NCI-H209 and NCI-H128) whereas insignificant binding reactions were observed for auto-

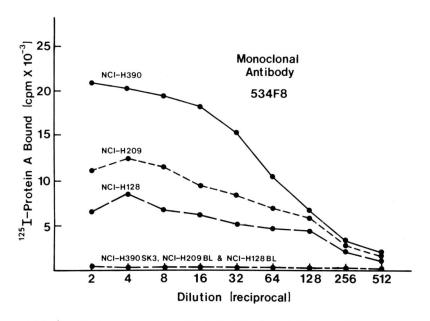

Figure 2. Titration binding curve using antibody 534F8 culture fluid on six different target plates as indicated. Points represent quadruplicate determinations. The three SCLC lines NCI-H390, NCI-H209, and NCI-H128 (derived from different patients) showed significant antibody binding. However, the autologous non-SCLC target cell lines (skin fibroblast NCI-H390SK3 and B-lymphoblastoid NCI-H209BL and NCI-H128BL) failed to demonstrate antibody binding.

logous skin fibroblast line NCI-H390SK3 and autologous B-lymphoblastoid cells (NCI-H128BL, NCI-H209BL) derived from the same patients donating the SCLC tumor. These findings support the existence of a common antigenic expression among SCLC lines and the lack of that expression on autologous nonmalignant cell lines.

To verify that the SCLC selective monoclonal antibodies were not recognizing an antigenic product of *in vitro* cultivation, it was critical to demonstrate that such antibodies would react with small cell tumor samples taken directly from patients without intervening culture. Toward this end we have used a direct immune detection assay, employing ^{125}I-labeled monoclonal antibodies, to evaluate the potential usefulness of these reagents as a diagnostic tool for SCLC. Table 2 shows the binding reaction of iodinated mouse antibody 534F8 and rat antibody 600D11 on necropsy samples of tumor-bearing and normal organs taken from SCLC and nontumorous patients. These reagents clearly discriminate tissue specimens having SCLC involvement from those samples which lack the tumor. Necropsy tissue of several organs harvested from donors without malignant disease failed to show significant binding with the exception of kidney. The latter reaction is currently under investigation to better define whether this represents specific or nonspecific binding.

4. IMMUNE-HISTOCHEMICAL DETECTION OF SCLC

Monoclonal antibodies can be used for the immune-histochemical stain-

Table 2. Direct radioimmune detection of ^{125}I labeled monoclonal antibody binding to small cell lung cancer necropsy specimens.

Specimen	Binding ratio[c]	
	^{125}I-534F8[a]	^{125}I-600D11[b]
Small cell lung cancer cell lines	33–78	15–48
B-lymphoblastoid cell lines	<2	<2
Small cell lung cancer tumor specimens from lung or liver	20–55	25–48
Normal lung (small cell lung cancer patient)	<2	<2
Normal liver (small cell lung cancer patient)	<2	<2
Normal tissue from necropsy: brain, spleen, muscle, colon, gall bladder, urinary bladder, and prostate	<2	<2

[a] Mouse IgM kappa (anti-SCLC).
[b] Rat IgM kappa (anti-SCLC).
[c] Binding ratio = cpm test minus cpm background divided by cpm background.

ing of SCLC in pathological specimens. We have demonstrated this capability, on paraffin embedded tissue, using antibody 534F8 in combination with biotinylated horse antimouse IgG and an avidin-biotin-peroxidase complex (ABC) [16, 36]. Figure 3c represents the immune localization of SCLC foci in liver metastases. Interestingly, the more diffuse infiltrates of SCLC were not discernible by immunochemical staining, thus illustrating the heterogeneity of tumor antigen expression found within a given patient.

5. IMMUNE RECOGNITION OF SCLC ANTIGENIC DETERMINANTS ON OTHER HUMAN TUMOR TYPES

Immune histopathological typing of human tumors can readily be accomplished with the use of monoclonal antibodies. We have extensively evaluated those monoclonal antibodies isolated by our screening strategy against

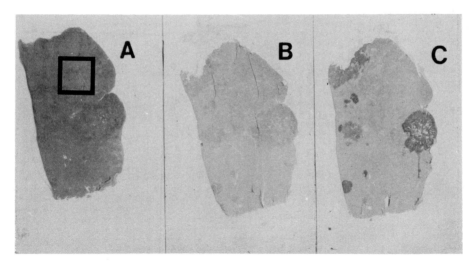

Figure 3. Composite picture representing the immune histochemical staining of necropsy slice of liver involved with metastatic SCLC. Serial section (A) H & E stain; (B) complete immune reaction minus monoclonal antibody 534F8; (C) complete immune reaction in the presence of antibody 534F8. The formalin fixed-paraffin embedded tissue specimen was processed for immune histochemical staining in the following manner: tissue sections were first deparaffinized in xylene and then exposed to a 1% bovine serum albumin solution (with or without monoclonal antibody 534F8), followed by sequential incubations in normal horse sera, biotinylated horse antimous IgG, avidin-biotin-peroxidase complex (Vector Laboratories, Burlingame, CA). Immune-enzyme deposition was then demonstrated using 0.01% hydrogen peroxide-0.05% diaminobensidine tetrahydrochloride. In serial section (C), several focal infiltrates of SCLC are clearly visible as dense nodules that exemplify immunochemical staining of tumor. However, the more diffuse infiltrates of tumor (identified as the boxed region of the H & E stain, section (A), lack immune depositions of stain and illustrate the existence of tumor heterogeneity within the same tissue section.

Table 3. Monoclonal antibody binding phenotypes to various tissue cultures lines.

Human cell lines	Binding phenotypes [a]		
	534F8 [b]	624A6 [c]	604A9 [c]
Small cell lung cancer	+	+	+
Adenocarcinoma	+	−	−
Squamous cell carcinoma	+	−	−
Large cell carcinoma	−	−	−
Melanoma	−	−	−
Glioblastoma	−	−	−
Osteogenic sarcoma	−	−	−
Breast cancer	+	+	+
Neuroblastoma	+	+	−
B cell lymphomas	−	−	−
T cell lymphomas	−	−	−

[a] (+) = binding ratio > 5; (−) = binding ratio < 2.
[b] Mouse IgM kappa antibody.
[c] Rat IgM kappa antibody.

a variety of other human tumor types. These reagents can be used to score tumors based on antigenic expression. As exemplified in Table 3, antibodies 534F8, 624A6, and 604A9 identify three distinct antigenic determinants present on SCLC and showing selective expression on other tumor types. Such information has revealed an unsuspected interrelationship between lung cancer and other human tumors. At present it is not known if SCLC arises from neural crest or endodermal structures [20]. Heteroantisera to SCLC detect antigenic determinants that fit both categories [37]. Interestingly, our monoclonal antibodies define three distinct antigenic determinants: 604A9 antigen unique to neural crest derivative (neuroblastoma), 624A6 antigen expressed on both neural crest and ectodermally (breast cancer) derived tumors, and 534F8 antigen present on neural crest, ectodermal and endodermal (adenocarcinoma) derivatives.

6. MONOCLONAL ANTIBODIES SELECTIVE FOR SCLC: POTENTIAL DIAGNOSTIC AND THERAPEUTIC USE

We have reviewed the technology employed for the generation and characterization of SCLC selective monoclonal antibodies. These reagents show preferential binding to many SCLC tissue culture lines and SCLC necropsy samples but failed to react with a variety of autologous cell lines and normal tissues. We have demonstrated that such reagents can be used in the immu-

Table 4. Potential clinicial applications of monoclonal antibodies.

Diagnostic use:
  Immunohistopathology
  Early detection of antigens
  Early detection of antigens
  Nuclear medicine imaging
  Predictor of prognosis
  Predictor of response to therapy

Therapeutic use:
  Direct cytotoxicity
    Antibody-dependent cellular cytotoxicity
    Complement mediated cytotoxicity
  Adjuvant cytotoxicity
    Drug, toxin, and cell conjugates
    Radionuclide conjugates
    Radiofocusing (boron conjugated antibody)
  Growth inhibition
  Specific binding of drug loaded liposomes
  Ex vivo therapy of bone marrow
  Regulation of immunity

nohistochemical staining of patients' specimens. Furthermore, these antibodies have been utilized in the immune histological typing of human tumors and have defined antigenic determinants which will aid in assigning embryologic origin.

Prospective applications for the clinical use of monoclonal antibodies as diagnostic and therapeutic reagents of lung cancer are summarized in Table 4. As with any other therapeutic drug, the antitumor monoclonal antibodies must undergo a series of clinical trials (Phase I and Phase II) to validate absence of toxicity and efficacy of the reagent. These antibodies can be used for evaluating the clinical status of patients: imaging studies using isotope-labeled antibodies [38, 39] can assess the extent of tumor involvement and measure the effectiveness of routine therapy (decrease in tumor size); detection of circulating antigen can be used as a diagnostic indicator or be correlated to the response of routine therapy [40]. Of potential therapeutic value in the treatment of lung cancer are those monoclonal antibodies which have direct cytotoxic effects on pulmonary malignancies. This type of approach to neoplastic therapy has already been utilized in the treatment of lymphoma-leukemia [41–45]. Ancillary reagents used for increasing the killing potency of monoclonal antibodies include conjugating drugs, toxins, radionuclides, or polymorphonuclear leukocytes, and the use of antibody specificity to target therapy [46–48]. Monoclonal antibodies can convey tumor cell specificity to liposomes containing cytotoxic drugs [49]. Boron

34

can be conjugated to tumor-specific antibodies and when excited by external radiation will emit low energy particles capable of killing tumor cells. Monoclonal antibodies with specificity for T cell subsets may be used to regulate antitumor immunity. Finally, there is the use of tumor-specific antibodies in *ex vivo* therapy of bone marrow. Autologous bone marrow transplants have been used to rescue a patient following a lethal dose of chemoradiotherapy. Monoclonal antibodies could be used to clean up bone marrows contaminated with small amounts of tumor cells prior to reinfusing the patient. All of these clinical applications await the isolation and characterization of antibodies with sufficient tumor selectivity and the design of appropriate clinical trials.

REFERENCES

1. Kohler G, Milstein C: Continuous cultures of fused cells secreting antibody of predefined specificity. Nature 256:495–497, 1975.
2. Kennett RH, Gilbert F: Hybrid myelomas producing antibodies against a human neuroblastoma antigen present on fetal brain. Science 203:1120–1121, 1979.
3. Schregg JF, Diserens AC, Carrel S, Accolia RS, de Tribolet N: Human glioma-associated antigens detected by monoclonal antibodies. Cancer Res 41:1209–1213, 1981.
4. Herlyn M, Steplewski Z, Herlyn D, Koprowski H: Colorectal carcinoma-specific antigen: detection by means of monoclonal antibodies. Proc Natl Acad Sci USA 76:1438–1442, 1979.
5. Koprowski H, Steplewski Z, Mitchell K, Herlyn M, Herlyn D, Fuhrer P: Colorectal carcinoma antigens detected by hybridoma antibodies. Somatic Cell Genet 5:957–972, 1979.
6. Magnani JL, Brochkaus M, Smith DF, Ginsburg U, Blasczyk M, Mitchell KF, Steplewski Z, Koprowski H: A monosialoganglioside is a monoclonal antibody-defined antigen of colon carcinoma. Science 212:55–56, 1981.
7. Schlom J, Wunderlich D, Teramoto YA: Generation of human monoclonal antibodies reactive with human mammary carcinoma cells. Proc Natl Acad Sci USA 77:6841–6845, 1980.
8. Nadler LM, Stashenko P, Hardy R, Schlossman SF: A monoclonal antibody defining a lymphoma-associated antigen in man. J Immunol 125:570–577, 1980.
9. Levy R, Dilley J, Fox RI, Warnke R: A human thymus-leukemia antigen defined by hybridoma monoclonal antibodies. Proc Natl Acad Sci USA 76:6552–6556, 1979.
10. Rite J, Pesando JM, Notis-McConarty J, Lazarus H, Schlossman SF: A monoclonal antibody to human acute lymphoblastic leukaemia antigen. Nature 283:583–585, 1980.
11. Koprowski H, Steplewski Z, Herlyn D, Herlyn M: Study of antibodies against human melanoma produced by somatic cell hybrids. Proc Natl Acad Sci USA 75:3405–3409, 1978.
12. Imai K, Ng A, Ferrone S: Characterization of monoclonal antibodies to human melanoma-associated antigens. J Natl Cancer Inst 66:489–496, 1981.
13. Yeh MY, Hellstrom I, Brown JP, Warner GA, Hansen JA, Hellstrom RE: Cell surface antigens of human melanoma identified by monoclonal antibody. Proc Natl Acad Sci USA 76:2927–2931, 1979.
14. Dippold WG, Lloyd KO, Li LTC, Ikeda H, Oettgen HF, Old LJ: Cell surface antigens of human malignant melanoma: definition of six antigenic systems with mouse monoclonal antibodies. Proc Natl Acad Sci USA 77:6114–6118, 1980.

15. Cuttitta F, Rosen S, Gazdar AF, Minna JD: Monoclonal antibodies which demonstrate specificity for several types of human lung cancer. Proc Natl Acad Sci USA 78:4591–4595, 1981.

16. Minna JD, Cuttitta F, Rosen S, et al.: Methods for production of monoclonal antibodies with specificity for human lung cancer cells. In vitro 17:1058–1070, 1981.

17. Mazauric T, Mitchell KF, Letchworth GJ, Koprowski H, Steplewski Z: Monoclonal antibody-defined human lung cell surface protein antigens. Cancer Res 42:150–154, 1982.

18. Brenner BG, Jothy S, Shuster J, Fuks A: Monoclonal antibodies to human lung tumor antigens. Cancer Res 1982 (in press).

19. Minna JD, Higgins GA, Glatstein EJ: Cancer of the lung. In: Principles and Practice of Oncology. DeVita VT, et al. (eds). Philadelphia: JB Lippincott, 1981, pp 396–473.

20. Gazdar AF, Carney DN, Guccion JG, Baylin SB: Small cell carcinoma of the lung: cellular origin and relationship to other pulmonary tumors. In: Small Cell Lung Cancer. Greco FA, et al. (eds). New York: Grune & Stratton, 1981, pp 145–175.

21. Matthews MJ, Gordon PR: Morphology and pleural malignancies. In: Lung – Clinical Diagnosis and Treatment. Strauss MJ, (ed). New York: Grune & Stratton, 1977, pp 49–69.

22. Matthews MJ, Gazdar AF: Pathology of small cell carcinoma of the lung and its subtypes: a clinico-pathologic correlation. In: Lung Cancer – Advances in Research and Treatment. Livingston RB, (ed). The Hague: Martinus Nijhoff, 1981, pp 283–306.

23. Gazdar AF, Carney DN, Guccion JG, et al.: Expression of ultrastructural, biochemical, immunological and cytogenetic markers in cell lines of small cell carcinoma of the lung and its morphological variants (submitted for publication).

24. Gazdar AF, Carney DN, Russell EK, et al.: Establishment of continuous clonable cultures of small-cell carcinoma of the lung which have amine precursor uptake and decarboxylation cell properties. Cancer Res 40:3502–3507, 1980.

25. Carney DN, Gazdar AF, Minna JD: Positive correlation between histological tumor involvement and generation of tumor cell colonies in agarose in specimens taken directly from patients with small-cell carcinoma of the lung. Cancer Res 40:1820–1823, 1980.

26. Simms E, Gazdar AF, Abrams PG, et al.: Growth of human small cell (oat cell) carcinoma of the lung in serum-free growth factor supplemented medium. Cancer Res 40:4356–4363, 1980.

27. Carney DN, Bunn PA, Gazdar AF, et al.: Selective growth in serum-free hormone-supplemented medium of tumor cells obtained by biopsy from patients with small cell carcinoma of the lung. Proc Natl Acad Sci USA 78:3185–3189, 1981.

28. Gazdar AF, Zweig MH, Carney DN, et al.: Level of creatine-kinase and its BB isoenzyme in lung cancer specimens and cultures. Cancer Res 41:2773–2777, 1981.

29. Moody TW, Pert CB, Gazdar AF, et al.: High levels of intracellular bombesin characterize human small-cell lung carcinoma. Science 214:1246–1248, 1981.

30. Radice PA, Dermody WC: Clonal heterogeneity of hormone production by continuous cultures of small cell carcinoma of the lung (SCCL). Proc Am Assoc Cancer Res 21:41, 1980.

31. Whang-Peng J, Kao-Shan CS, Lee FC, et al.: A specific chromosomal defect associated with human small cell lung cancer: deletion 3p (14–23). Science 215:181–182, 1982.

32. Kearney JF, Radbruch A, Liesegang B: A new mouse myeloma cell line that has lost immunoglobulin expression but permits the construction of antibody-secreting hybrid cell lines. J. Immunol 123:1548-1550, 1979.

33. Galfre G, Howe SC, Milstein C, et al.: Antibodies to major histocompatibility antigens produced by hybrid cell lines. Nature 266:550-552, 1977.

34. Kennett RH, Denis KA, Tung AS, Klinman NR: Hybrid plasmacytoma production: fusions

with adult spleen cells, monoclonal spleen fragments, neonatal spleen cells and human spleen cells. Curr Top Microbiol Immunol 81:77–91, 1978.

35. Nowinski RC, Lostrom ME, Tam MR, *et al.*: The isolation of hybrid cell lines producing monoclonal antibodies against the p15(E) protein of ecotropic murine leukemia viruses. Virology 93:111–126, 1979.

36. Hsu SM, Raine L, Fanger H: The use of avidin-biotin-peroxidase complex (ABC) in immunoperoxidase techniques: a comparison between ABC and unlabeled antibody (PAP) procedures. J Histochem Cytochem 29:577–581, 1981.

37. Bell CE, Seetharam S, McDaniel RC: Endodermally-derived and neural crest-derived differentiation antigens expressed by a human lung tumor. J Immunol 116:1236–1243, 1976.

38. Scheinberg DA, Strand M, Gansow OA: Tumor imaging with radioactive metal chelates conjugated to monoclonal antibodies. Science 215:1511–1513, 1982.

39. Ballou B, Levine G, Hakala TR, Solter S: Tumor location detected with radioactively labeled monoclonal antibody and external scintigraphy. Science 206:844–847, 1979.

40. Koprowski H, Herlyn M, Steplewski Z, Sears HF: Specific antigen in serum of patients with colon carcinoma. Science 212:53–55, 1981.

41. Nadler LM, Stashenko P, Hardy P, *et al.*: Serotherapy of a patient with a monoclonal antibody directed against a human lymphoma-associated antigen. Cancer Res 40:3147–3154, 1980.

42. Ritz J, Pesando JM, Sallan SE, *et al.*: Serotherapy of acute lymphoblastic leukemia with monoclonal antibody. Blood 58:141–152, 1981.

43. Miller RA, Maloney DG, McKillop J, Levy R: *In vivo* effects of murine hybridoma monoclonal antibody in a patient with T-cell leukemia. Blood 58:78–86, 1981.

44. Miller RA, Levy R: Response to cutaneous T-cell lymphoma to therapy with hybridoma monoclonal antibody. Lancet 2:226–228, 1981.

45. Miller RA, Maloney DG, Warnke R, Levy R: Treatment of B-cell lymphoma with monoclonal anti-idiotype antibody. N Engl J Med 306: 517–522, 1982.

46. Olsnes S: Directing toxins to cancer cells. Nature 290:84, 1981.

47. Scheinberg DA, Strand M: Leukemic cell targeting and therapy by monoclonal antibody in a mouse model system. Cancer Res 42:44–49, 1982.

48. Belles-Isles M, Page M: Anti-oncofoetal proteins for targeting cytotoxic drugs. Int J Immunopharmacol 3:97–102, 1981.

49. Leserman LD, Machy P, Barbet J: Cell-specific drug transfer from liposomes bearing monoclonal antibodies. Nature 293:226–228, 1981.

3. Transforming Growth Factors (TGFs) and Human Lung Cancer Cells

STEPHEN A. SHERWIN and GEORGE J. TODARO

1. INTRODUCTION

Growth factors are substances which stimulate cell division in a variety of target tissues [1, 2]. Such factors include low molecular weight polypeptides such as epidermal growth factor, platelet-derived growth factor, fibroblast growth factor, and the insulin growth factors, and relatively higher molecular weight glycoproteins such as colony stimulatory factors, which act primarily on hematopoietic stem cells [3–8]. There is increasing evidence that growth factors play a role in normal embryogenesis as well as in the regeneration of normal tissues in the adult [1]. Moreover, it has recently been observed that human tumor cells of various types are capable of producing biologically active peptide growth factors and it has been postulated that these factors promote or support the growth of the very same tumor cells which produce them [9–11]. This phenomenon, which may be characteristic of many cells, has been termed 'autocrine secretion' [12] and to the extent that growth factors produced by tumor cells are necessary for the survival of those cells *in vivo*, new approaches to cancer treatment could possibly involve the use of appropriate 'antigrowth factor' substances. This chapter will examine in detail the association between one class of peptide growth factors, transforming growth factors (TGFs), and human lung cancer and will address the potential clinical applications of these observations.

2. TRANSFORMING GROWTH FACTORS

Transforming growth factors (TGFs) are low molecular weight polypeptides which can promote anchorage-independent growth in semi-solid medium of a variety of nontransformed and transformed cells [11, 13–14]. The ability of cells to grow as colonies in soft agar-containing medium is a well-

Greco, FA (ed), Biology and Management of Lung Cancer. ISBN 0-89838-554-7.
© *1983, Martinus Nijhoff Publishers, Boston. Printed in The Netherlands.*

recognized property of the transformed phenotype [15–17]. TGFs and related growth stimulatory peptides have been identified in serum-free culture supernatants of virally and chemically transformed rodent cells [13, 14, 18] and human tumor cells [11], cell extracts of virus and carcinogen-induced rodent tumors [19–21], embryonic rodent tissues [22], and most recently in the urine of patients with various types of disseminated cancer [23, 24]. To date, several TGF activities have been partially purified and characterized biochemically. The activities appear to reside in several molecular species of relatively low molecular weight (MW) (between 7,000 and 30,000) which are heat and acid-stable but sensitive to reducing agents and to proteases [11, 13]. Although immunologically non-crossreactive with epidermal growth factor (EGF), some (but not all) TGFs can compete with EGF for binding to its cell membrane receptor and are therefore thought to be, at least in part, functionally related to EGF. The ability of certain TGFs to bind to EGF receptors and thereby prevent their detection in radioreceptor assays, proved to be important in identifying those human tumor cells which were EGF receptor-negative and producers of relatively higher amounts of TGF [13]. More recently, a second class of TGFs has been identified which do not compete with EGF for binding to its receptor and which are potentiated by EGF in the soft agar growth factor assay [19–20]. These EGF-dependent TGFs do not produce morphologic transformation in the absence of EGF and have thus far been found in both normal and neoplastic rodent cells [19, 20].

Virally transformed rodent cell lines were the first cell type shown to produce factors capable of stimulating soft agar growth of nontransformed indicator cells [13, 14]. The initial observation of this phenomenon followed from earlier experiments which showed that these cells lacked EGF receptors and therefore might be producing EGF-related growth factors which could bind to and mask membrane EGF receptors. Murine 3T3 cells transformed by Moloney sarcoma virus (MSV) were tested initially since these cells were EGF receptor-negative in contrast to DNA virus (polyoma) or chemically (methylcholanthrene) transformed cells which were EGF receptor-positive [25, 26]. Serum-free culture supernatants from MSV-transformed 3T3 cells were extracted with 1 M acetic acid, lyophilized and chromatographed on a Bio-Gel® P-60 system. Column fractions were then tested for mitogenic (growth-promoting) activity as measured by thymidine incorporation, EGF-competing activity, and soft agar growth factor activity as measured by the ability to stimulate colony growth of nontransformed normal rat kidney (NRK) fibroblasts. These experiments revealed three major peaks of activity with apparent MWs of 7,000, 12,000 and 25,000. All three of these different molecular species demonstrated, in nanogram concentrations, both mitogenic and soft agar growth-promoting activity, as well as EGF-competing activity. However, these activities were distinguishable from EGF itself by virtue of molecular weight differences, the ability to stimulate soft agar growth, and a lack of immunologic crossreactivity with EGF. The EGF-related soft agar growth-promoting activity was termed 'sarcoma growth factor' or SGF since the 3T3 cells producing them had been transformed by a sarcoma virus. SGFs have since been identified in the culture supernatants of other virally-transformed rodent cells including Abelson murine leukemia virus transformed fibroblasts [27]. The discovery of SGFs led directly to the subsequent identification of the closely related transforming growth factors (TGFs) in supernatant fluids and cell extracts of rodent cells transformed by agents other than RNA sarcoma viruses, as well as various human carcinomas and sarcomas. The ability of TGFs to reversibly stimulate soft agar growth of nontransformed cells and thereby reversibly induce the transformed phenotype is the characteristic property of this class of peptide growth factors.

Following the isolation of SGFs in the supernatants of MSV sarcoma virus-transformed murine cells, TGFs with similar properties were identified in biochemical extracts of these cells following acid-ethanol extraction and Bio-Gel® P-60 chromatography [21]. Such intracellular TGFs resemble their extracellular counterparts with regard to molecular weight and other biochemical properties, as well as their ability to stimulate soft agar growth of phenotypically normal cells. These observations further support the hypothesis that the TGF activity detected in the culture supernatants of the virally transformed cells was, in fact, produced by these cells and subsequently released into the culture medium. The same biochemical extraction procedure was also applied to the analysis of a chemically-induced murine bladder tumor and a similar TGF activity was identified [21]. This suggests that the production of molecules with the properties of TGFs or SGFs is not unique to virally-induced tumors. In fact, acid-ethanol extraction of whole mouse embryos (10–12 days old) followed by Bio-Gel® P-10 chromatography has recently been shown to detect TGF activity. This indicates that functionally related molecules can also be found in certain nonneoplastic fetal tissues, suggesting that TGFs of one type or another may play a role in some aspect of normal embryogenesis [22].

Further analysis of TGFs isolated from virally and chemically transformed rodent cells have shown that a certain degree of heterogeneity exists among TGF molecules. It now appears that there are at least two different types of TGF activities: (1) that which competes with EGF for binding to its receptor and is not potentiated by EGF in the soft agar growth factor assay, and (2) that which does not compete with EGF for receptor binding but is potentiated by EGF in the soft agar colony assay. Both types of TGF activity have recently been identified in serum-free culture supernatants and biochemical extracts of various transformed rodent cells [18–20]. In addition, the TGF activity which does not bind to the EGF receptor has been identified in extracts of the submaxillary gland and other normal tissues of the adult mouse [20]. Indeed, there is growing evidence that both types of TGF activity can also be identified in human tumor cells.

As note above, TGF activity of the sort initially described for rodent tumor cells has since been detected in serum-free supernatants collected from certain human tumor cell lines [11]. The human tumors first tested were those cell lines found to be lacking EGF receptors in a radiolabelled EGF binding assay. Three cell lines derived from specimens of melanoma, bronchogenic carcinoma, and rhabdomyosarcoma and found to be EGF receptor-negative were grown in serum-free medium. Culture supernatants were extracted with 1 M acetic acid and chromatographed on a Bio-Gel® P-100 system using methodology similar to that developed for the rodent SGF analysis discussed previously [13]. Figure 1 shows the results of experiments in which culture supernatants from the human rhabdomyosarcoma cell line A673 were tested for soft agar growth-promoting (TGF) and EGF-competing activity. One major peak of TGF activity was identified with an

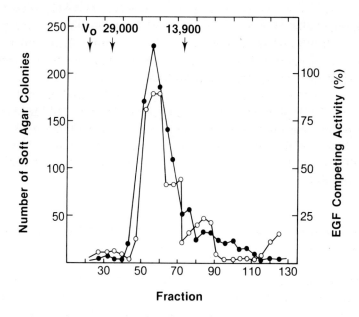

Figure 1. Bio-Gel® P-100 chromatography of 1 *M* acetic acid-extracted culture supernatants from A673 rhabdomyosarcoma cells. Column fractions were assayed for soft agar growth factor activity as determined by colony growth of NRK cells (●) and for EGF-competing activity in a radioreceptor assay using radiolabelled mouse EGF and A431 human carcinoma cells (○). Column markers were carbonic anhydrase (MW29,000) and RNAse (MW13,900) and the void is designated by V_0.

Table 1. A comparison of human TGF and mouse EGF.

	TGF	EGF
Molecular weight	7,400–30,000	6,000
Mitogenic activity	+	+
Ability to bind to EGF receptors	+	+
Soft agar growth-promoting activity	+	−
Reactivity with antibody to EGF	−	+

apparent MW of approximately 20,000 and this coincided with the major peak of EGF-competing activity. However, when this TGF activity was further analyzed by carboxymethylcellulose chromatography it was separated into two components: a major peak which had EGF-competing activity and a minor peak which did not. Thus, TGF activities of two types, both related and unrelated to EGF and perhaps similar to the two types described for rodent tumors [19, 20], can also be identified in human tumors.

The TGF activity found in serum-free culture supernatants of human tumor cells is in some respects similar to the TGFs and SGFs described for rodent tumor cells. Human TGFs are also heat- and acid-stable polypeptides which like EGF are potent mitogens but unlike EGF can reversibly stimulate soft agar growth of nontransformed cells, thereby reversibly inducing the transformed phenotype. Moreover, TGF from human tumors is further distinguished from murine and human EGF based on its amino acid composition. TGF obtained from the human melanoma cell line A2058 and purified by reverse phase high pressure liquid chromatography lacks both tyrosine and methionine, thus distinguishing it from both murine and human EGF [28]. Table 1 compares some of the properties of human TGF and murine EGF.

3. TRANSFORMING GROWTH FACTOR ACTIVITY AND HUMAN LUNG CANCER CELLS

Among the EGF receptor-negative human tumor cell lines tested for TGF activity in the experiments described above is the bronchogenic carcinoma cell line 9812. This cell line, derived from a large cell anaplastic carcinoma, produced an EGF-related TGF activity of approximately 20,000 MW which is capable of reversibly stimulating soft agar colony growth of nontransformed indicator cells [11]. Analysis of serum-free culture supernatants from 9812 cells using the same methodology described for A673 rhabdomyosarcoma cells identified peaks of NRK colony stimulating activity and

EGF-competing activity at approximately the 20,000 MW fractions of a Bio-Gel® P-100 chromatography system.

In order to determine if TGF production correlated with a lack of detectable EGF receptors or if, in fact, EGF receptor-positive cell lines could produce TGF activities, a survey of 15 well-characterized human lung cancer cell lines was undertaken [29–31]. These cell lines included 9 derived from small cell carcinoma specimens, 3 of which were termed 'converters' because they had lost the specific morphologic and biochemical features of small cell carcinoma cell lines after prolonged passage *in vitro* [29, 32]. The other 6 lines were derived from non-small cell carcinoma specimens including 3 adenocarcinomas, 1 epidermoid carcinoma, and 2 large cell carcinomas. All 15 cell lines were tested for their ability to bind radiolabelled EGF to cell membrane receptors and for their ability to stimulate NRK cells to grow as colonies in agar using previously described methods [33]. The

Table 2. EGF receptors and TGF production by human lung cancer cell lines.

Cell line	EGF bound fmol/10^6 cells [a]	NRK colonies/10^3 cells at 5 days [b]
Non small cell		
U1752 (epidermoid)	64.0	240
NCI-H157 (large cell)	27.1	310
9812 (large cell)	<0.1	355
A549 (bronchioalveolar)	23.4	305
NCI-H123 (adenocarcinoma)	8.8	165
NCI-H125 (adenocarcinoma)	7.8	210
Small cell		
NCI-H69	<0.1	215
NCI-H128	<0.1	150
NCI-H146	<0.1	55
NCI-H175	<0.1	190
NCI-H187	<0.1	235
NCI-N231	<0.1	80
Small cell converter		
NCI-H82	<0.1	60
NCI-N177	<0.1	100
NCI-N417	4.5	0

[a] Bound EGF was determined by incubating a suspension of 10^6 cells with 2.5 ng of ^{125}I-labelled mouse EGF, washing the cells, and calculating bound radioactivity. Nonspecific binding as determined by coincubation with an excess of 2.5 μg of unlabelled EGF was subtracted in each case.

[b] Lung cancer cell lines were used as feeder layers under a base of 0.5% agar-containing media. NRK colonies greater than 6 cells in a 0.3% agar overlay were scored in 4 high power fields after 5 days of incubation.

results of these experiments are shown in Table 2. Small cell and non-small cell human lung cancer cell lines are markedly different with respect to the presence or absence of EGF receptors. Non-small cell cultures have EGF receptors which are easily detected whereas small cell cultures uniformly lack these receptors. One of three small cell 'converters' had detectable EGF receptors, thus suggesting that during prolonged passage *in vitro* the appearance of measurable EGF receptors may accompany the loss of the specific morphological and biochemical markers associated with small cell cultures. The differences between small cell and non-small cell lung cancer cell lines with regard to the presence or absence of EGF receptors are not unique to this class of membrane receptor. In another series of experiments reported previously [33], these same cell lines were also shown to differ with regards to the distribution of cell membrane receptors for nerve growth factor (NGF). NGF receptors were detected at low levels on 3 of 6 small cell cultures and on all 3 small cell converters, but none of 6 non-small cell cultures. Thus, the two major groups of lung cancer, small cell and non-small cell, differ markedly with regards to the distribution of cell membrane receptors for at least two of the peptide growth factors, EGF and NGF.

Table 2 also shows the results of the experiments in which the 15 human lung cancer cell lines were tested for their ability to produce TGFs as measured by stimulation of NRK cells to grow as colonies in agar. In these experiments the various human lung cancer cell lines were used as feeder layers in 0.5% agar and overlaid with 0.3% agar containing a suspension of NRK cells. NRK colonies were scored at 5 days. As shown in Table 2, all but one of the 15 human lung cancer cell lines were capable of stimulating the soft agar growth of NRK. These results include all 6 non-small cell lines, 5 of which have easily detectable EGF receptors. Similar observations were made, although with lower levels of activity, using small volumes of conditioned medium from these lung cancer cell lines. It would appear, therefore, that the production of TGFs, as measured in this fashion, does not correlate with the presence or absence of EGF receptors, but rather that the production of TGFs appears to be a very general property of human lung cancer cells growing *in vitro*. The TGFs produced by various human lung cancer cell lines have yet to be characterized biochemically, except for the factors produced by the bronchogenic carcinoma cell line which were described above. The TGF activities produced by this EGF receptor negative cell line are of the type capable of binding to the EGF receptor. It remains to be seen whether TGFs produced by EGF receptor positive non-small cell lung cancer cultures resemble the non-EGF related TGFs recently identified in transformed rodent cells [19, 20]. On the other hand, it is possible that all lung cancer cell lines may produce more than one type of TGF activity.

44

4. TRANSFORMING GROWTH FACTOR ACTIVITY IN THE URINE OF PATIENTS WITH LUNG CANCERS AND OTHER CANCERS

Since nearly all human lung cancer cell lines examined were found to produce TGFs whether or not they were EGF receptor-negative, it seemed reasonable to examine patients with various types of lung cancer for *in vivo* evidence of TGF production by their tumor. As noted previously, TGFs are low molecular weight, acid-stable polypeptides, and therefore might be expected to be recoverable from the urine. In preliminary experiments [24], 1–2 liter quantities of urine were collected from a patient with small cell lung cancer and an appropriate normal control. These urines were extracted with acid-ethanol and were subsequently analyzed on a Bio-Gel® P-100 chromatography system. Column fractions were then assayed according to the usual methods for TGF soft agar growth-promoting activity and EGF

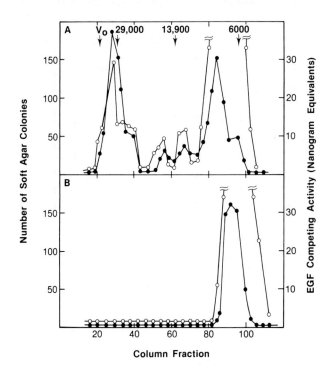

Figure 2. Bio-Gel® P-100 chromatography of acid-ethanol extracted urine from: (A) a patient with small cell lung cancer, and (B) a normal male. Column fractions were assayed for soft agar growth factor activity against NRK cells (●) and for EGF-competing activity in a radioreceptor assay using A431 human carcinoma cells (○). Column markers were carbonic anhydrase (MW29,000) RNAse (MW13,900) and insulin (MW6,000). The column void is indicated by V_0.

competing activity. The results of this experiment are shown in Figure 2. Both the small cell lung cancer patient's urine and the normal control's urine had evidence of TGF activity in the 6,000–8,000 MW range. However, the lung cancer patient's urine also had evidence of a higher molecular weight TGF activity at MW 30,000–35,000, as well as two minor activities at MW 10,000 and 20,000. Figure 2 also shows that the peak of EGF competing activity for the high molecular weight TGF coincides with the peak of soft agar growth-promoting activity and, in fact, further purification of this activity by high pressure liquid chromatography indicates that these two activities coelute. In contrast, EGF competing activity and TGF activity in the 6,000–8,000 MW range appear not to coelute and the relationship between these two activities is yet to be defined. It is possible that this low molecular weight TGF activity in normal urine corresponds to the non-EGF related TGF activity found in normal rodent cells which requires the presence of EGF for the expression of its soft agar growth promoting activi-

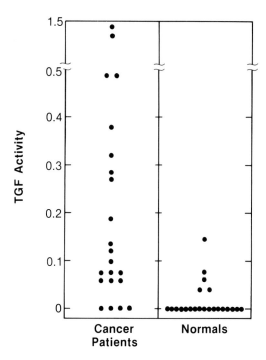

Figure 3. TGF activity in the urine of cancer patients and normal controls (including nonmalignant inflammatory disease patients) following chromatography of acid-extracted urine on Bio-Gel® P-30. Results are expressed as a ratio of high molecular weight TGF activity (MW30,000–35,000) to low molecular weight TGF activity (MW6,000–8,000), so as to correct for the variability in the NRK colony assay. For each urine tested, colonies greater than 6 cells were scored in the 3 peak fractions of each molecular weight region.

ty [19, 20]. It is likewise possible that the soft agar growth stimulatory properties of the low molecular weight urinary TGF activity depends on the presence of EGF in normal human urine, a substance sometimes referred to as 'urogastrone' [5].

In order to determine whether the high molecular weight TGF (MW 30–35,000) found in the small cell lung cancer patient's urine (but not in the normal control's) was tumor-associated a larger number of urines were collected from patients with a variety of disseminated cancers, as well as normal controls of comparable age and sex. These urines were tested using a scaled-down extraction method for the presence of the high molecular weight urinary TGF. Urines were extracted with 1 M acetic acid centrifuged to remove acid insoluble material, and chromatographed on Bio-Gel® P-30. TGF activity as measured in the NRK colony assay was then scored in both the 30–35,000 and 6–8,000 MW ranges for each urine tested. Figure 3 summarizes the results of these experiments. Since all urines tested including both cancer patients and normal controls were found to have TGF activity at MW 6–8,000, the data in Figure 3 is expressed as a ratio of TGF activity at MW 30–35,000 to TGF activity at MW 6–8,000 in order to control for the variability in the assay. Using this approach, 18 of 22 patients with a variety of disseminated cancers, including 2 of 2 patients with small cell lung cancer and 2 of 3 patients with non-small cell lung cancer, had detectable high molecular weight TGF activity in their urines. One of the 2 patients with small cell lung cancer was among the most positive of the urines tested with a TGF ratio of approximately 1.35. In contrast, only 5 of 22 of the normal controls had the activity in their urine and then only at fairly low concentrations. Taken together, these results indicate that while it may not be specific for patients with advanced cancer, the high molecular weight TGF activity found in the urine of patients with lung cancer and other types of cancer is clearly a tumor-associated activity. Although not yet firmly established, based on the experiments described which have shown that human lung cancer cells produce similar TGFs *in vitro*, it seems likely that the high molecular weight tumor-associated TGF activity found in the urine is a product of the patient's tumor and therefore has clear potential as a biologically active tumor marker. TGF production by human lung cancer cells is thus analogous to the ectopic production of polypeptide hormones including ACTH, ADH, and calcitonin by both small cell and non-small cell lung cancers [34, 35]. Unlike these hormones, however, the tumor-associated high molecular weight TGF may perhaps have the potential to act on the tumor cell producing it and thereby support its growth [10].

5. CONCLUSIONS

Transforming growth factors (TGFs) are a group of polypeptides which interact with the epidermal growth factor receptor and have the unique property of being able to stimulate the growth in soft agar of nontransformed indicator cells. TGFs, thus, have the ability to reversibly induce the transformed phenotype. The precise molecular mechanism by which these events take place is unknown. However, it has recently been shown that TGFs can phosphorylate tryosine residues in the EGF receptor and other membrane proteins in a fashion similar to the products of viral transforming genes and may therefore work through similar mechanisms [36]. Although TGF activities were originally detected in virally and chemically transformed rodent tumor cell extracts and culture supernatants they have also been identified and partially purified from human tumor cells. In this chapter, we have reviewed data to indicate that the vast majority of human lung cancer cells are producing TGFs whether or not they have detectable EGF receptors. Moreover, we have shown that these *in vitro* observations may correlate with the *in vivo* finding of tumor-associated higher molecular weight TGF activity in the urines of a high percentage of patients with disseminated cancers, including lung cancers and other cancers. Although initial experiments suggest that a decrease may occur following different forms of anticancer therapy, urinary TGF activity will clearly need to be further defined with regard to its value as a tumor marker that can be used to follow a patient's course and response to treatment. However, unlike other tumor markers now in use clinically, including carcinoembryonic antigen and alpha fetoprotein, urinary TGF has a well-defined biologic activity relating to the transformed phenotype and therefore may permit a more accurate assessment of the patient's malignancy. Finally, to the extent that the production of TGF and related molecules by tumor cells may be required for their survival *in vivo* (by means of what has been called 'autocrine secretion' [12]) the study of urinary TGF activity may allow the development of new approaches to cancer treatment involving the use of agents which can antagonize the effects of transforming growth factor activity.

REFERENCES

1. Golde DW, Herschman, HR, Aldens AJ, Groopman JE: Growth factors. Ann Intern Med 92:650-662, 1980.
2. Gospodarowicz D, Moran JS: Growth factors in mammalian cell culture. Ann. Rev Biochem 45:531-558, 1976.
3. Antoniades HN, Scher CD, Stiles DC: Purification of human platelet derived growth factor. Proc Natl Acad Sci 76:1809-1813, 1979.
4. Carpenter G, Cohen S: Epidermal growth factor. An Rev Biochem 48:193-216, 1979.

5. Cline MJ, Golde DW: Cellular interactions in hematopoiesis. Nature 277: 177–181, 1979.

6. Froesch ER, Zapf J, Rinderknecht E, Morell B, Schoenle E, Humble E: Insulin-like growth factor: Structure function and physiology. In: Cold Spring Harbor Conference on Cell Proliferation. Sato G, Ross R (eds). Cold Spring Harbor, New York: Cold Spring Harbor Press, 1979, Vol 6, pp 61–78.

7. Ross R, Glomset J, Kariya B, Harker L: A platelet-dependent serum factor that stimulates the proliferation of arterial smooth muscle cells *in vitro*. Proc Natl Acad Sci 71: 1207-1210, 1974.

8. Stanley ER, Hansen G, Woodcock J, Metcalf D: Colony stimulating factor and the regulation of granulopoiesis and macrophage production. Fed Proc 34: 2272–2278, 1975.

9. Todaro GJ, De Larco JE, Fryling C, Johnson PA, Sporn MB: Transforming growth factors (TGFs): Properties and possible mechanisms of action. J. Supramolec Struc and Cellular Biochem 15: 287–301, 1981.

10. Todaro GJ, De Larco JE, Marquardt H, Bryant ML, Sherwin SA, Sliski AH: Polypeptide growth factors produced by tumor cells and virus-transformed cells. In: Cold Spring Harbor Conferences on Cell Proliferation. Sato GH, Ross R (eds). Cold Spring Harbor, New York: Cold Spring Harbor Press, 1979, Vol 6, pp 113–127.

11. Todaro GJ, Fryling CM, De Larco JE: Transforming growth factors (TGFs) produced by certain human tumor cells: Polypeptides that interact with epidermal growth factor (EGF) receptors. Proc Natl Acad Sci 77:5258–5262, 1980.

12. Sporn MB, Todaro GJ: Autocrine secretion and malignant transformation of cells. New Engl J Med 303:878–880, 1980.

13. De Larco JE, Todaro GJ: Growth factors from murine sarcoma virus transformed cells. Proc Natl Acad Sci 75:4001–4005, 1978.

14. Todaro GJ, De Larco JE: Growth factors produced by sarcoma virus-transformed cells. Cancer Res 38:4147–4154, 1978.

15. Colburn NH, Bruegge WFV, Bates JR, Gray RH, Rossen JD, Delsey WH, Shimada T: Correlation of anchorage-independent growth with tumorigenicity of chemically transformed mouse epidermal cells. Cancer Res 38:624–634, 1978.

16. MacPherson I, Montagnier L: Agar suspension culture for selective assay of cells transformed by polyoma virus. Virology 23:291–294, 1964.

17. Shin S, Freedman VH, Risser R, Pollack R: Tumorigenicity of virus-transformed cells in nude mice is correlated specifically with anchorage independent growth *in vitro*. Proc Natl Acad Sci 72:4435–4439, 1975.

18. Moses HL, Branum EL, Proper JA, Robinson RA: Transforming growth factor production by chemically transformed cells. Cancer Res 41:2847–2848, 1981.

19. Roberts AB, Anzano MA, Lamb LC, Smith JM, Frolik CA, Marquardt H, Todaro GJ, Sporn MB: Isolation from murine sarcoma cells of a new class of transforming growth factors potentiated by epidermal growth factor. Nature 295:417–419, 1982.

20. Roberts AB, Anzano MA, Lamb LC, Smith JM, Sporn MB: New class of transforming growth factors potentiated by epidermal growth factor: isolation from neoplastic tissues. Proc Natl Acad Sci 78:5339–5343, 1981.

21. Roberts AB, Lamb LC, Newton DL, Sporn MB, De Larco JE, Todaro GJ: Transforming growth factors: Isolation of polypeptides from virally and chemically transformed cells by acid/ethanol extraction. Proc Natl Acad Sci 77:3494–3498, 1980.

22. Twardzik DR, Ranchalis JE, Todaro GJ: Mouse embryos contain transforming growth factors related to those isolated from tumor cells. Cancer Res 42:590–593, 1982.

23. Sherwin SA, Twardzik D, Bohn W, Cockley K, Todaro GJ: Tumor-associated transforming growth factor activity in the urine of patients with disseminated cancer. Cancer Res (in press).

24. Twardzik DR, Sherwin SA, Ranchalis JE, Todaro GJ: The urine of pregnant and tumor-bearing humans contains transforming growth factor 'likeb' activities. J. Natl Cancer Inst 69:793-798, 1982.

25. De Larco JE, Todaro GJ: Epithelioid and fibroblastic rat kidney cell clones: Epidermal growth factor (EGF) receptors and the effect of mouse sarcoma virus transformation. J Cell Physiol 94: 335-342, 1978.

26. Todaro GJ, De Larco JE, Cohen S: Transformation by murine and feline sarcoma viruses specifically blocks binding of epidermal growth factor to cells. Nature 264:26-31, 1976.

27. Twardzik DR, Todaro GJ, Marquardt H, Reynolds FH Jr, Stephenson JR: Abelson MuLV-induced transformation involves production of a polypeptide growth factor. Science 216: 894-897, 1982.

28. Marquardt H, Todaro GJ: Human transforming growth factor: Production by a melanoma cell line, purification, and initial characterization. J Biol Chem 257:5220-5225, 1982.

29. Gazdar AF, Carney DN, Russell EK, Sims EL, Baylin SB, Bunn PA, Guccion JG, Minna JD: Establishment of continuous, clonable tumorigenic lines of small cell carcinoma of the lung have amine precursor uptake and decarboxylation properties. Cancer Res 40: 3502-3507, 1980.

30. Giard DJ, Aaronson SA, Todaro GJ, Arnstein P, Kersey JM, Dosik H, Parks W: *In vitro* cultivation of human tumors: Establishment of cell lines derived from a series of solid tumors. J Natl Cancer Inst 51:1417-1423, 1973.

31. Lieber MM, Smith B, Szakal A, Nelson-Rees W, Todaro GJ: A continuous tumor cell line from a human lung cancer with properties of type II alveolar cells. Int J Cancer 17: 62-70, 1976.

32. Cohen MH, Matthews MJ: Small cell bronchogenic carcinoma: A distinct pathologic entity. Semin Oncol 5:234-243, 1978.

33. Sherwin SA, Minna JD, Gazdar AF, Todaro GJ: Expression of epidermal and nerve growth factor receptors and soft agar growth factor production by human lung cancer cells. Cancer Res 41: 3538-3542, 1981.

34. Gerwitz G, Yalow RS: Ectopic ACTH production in carcinoma of the lung. J Clin Invest 53: 1022-1032, 1974.

35. Silva OL, Becker KL, Primark A, Dappman JL, Snider RH: Ectopic secretion of calcitonin in oat-cell carcinoma. N Engl J Med 290:1122-1124, 1974.

36. Reynolds FH Jr, Todaro GJ, Fryling C, Stephenson JR: Human transforming growth factors induce tyrosine phosphorylation of EGF receptors. Nature 292: 259-262, 1981.

4. Tumor Cloning Assay: Application and Potential Usefulness in Lung Cancer Management

S. KENT CALLAHAN, CHARLES A. COLTMAN Jr., CLIFF KITTEN and

DANIEL D. VON HOFF

1. INTRODUCTION

The use of the clonogenic or stem-cell assay in clinical practice has demonstrated exponential growth over the past five years. An attempt will be made to outline the development of this system, including both practical and theoretical considerations. The current status of the assay in terms of its usefulness and its problems will be explored. In addition, the current data on correlations between *in vitro* results and clinical results will be presented. The last sections will be devoted to an analysis of one laboratory's data on the application of this system to patients with lung cancer. For further general considerations of the cloning assay, the reader is referred to recent comprehensive reviews of the system [1–4].

2. GENERAL DISCUSSION OF CLONOGENIC ASSAY

2.1. Stem cell concept

The stem-cell concept which has evolved from work on normal tissues such as the bone marrow and intestinal mucosa states that in every renewable tissue there exists a subpopulation of cells which can both reproduce themselves (self-renewal) as well as giving rise to a differentiating line of mature and functional cells [5]. In the marrow these stem cells are a very small proportion (1 %) of the total number of cells and in the intestine they have been found to occupy positions located only at the base of the crypts of Lieberkuhn [5]. The possibility that neoplasms contain a similar population of stem cells has been advanced as an attractive hypothesis. These tumor stem cells could be a very small percentage of the total number of tumor cells and may behave with different kinetics from most of the cells in the tumor. Again these cells would be characterized by both the ability for self-

Greco, FA (ed), Biology and Management of Lung Cancer. ISBN 0-89838-554-7.
© *1983, Martinus Nijhoff Publishers, Boston. Printed in The Netherlands.*

renewal as well as the ability to give rise to a large number of tumor cells which have lost this capacity for self-renewal. The detection of these 'stem cells' by their ability to produce colonies of tumor cells in the soft-agar system to be described below, and to evaluate their response to antineoplastic agents, forms the basis for the use of this *in vitro* system to aid in the treatment of patients with malignancies.

2.2. Historical considerations

In 1966 Bruce and his colleagues at the Ontario Cancer Institute, first demonstrated the possibility of studying stem cells from transplantable murine neoplasms by using a spleen colony assay [7]. Over the next ten years attempts to primarily culture human tumors to evaluate colony formation met with little success because of the inability to provide an environment which would give tumor cells a selective advantage over normal cells (particularly fibroblasts). The major breakthrough which circumvented this problem was made by Hamburger and Salmon [8, 9], who devised a soft-agar system capable of supporting growth of human myeloma cells. With the advent of this new technology, the culturing of human tumor stem cells has become a reality.

2.3. Methodology

The actual growing of tumor cell colonies requires a number of steps. These include: (1) preparation of a single cell suspension; (2) plating the cells in a system which will support their growth but inhibit the growth of unwanted nonmalignant cells; and (3) selection of proper conditions of drug exposure that will make the *in vitro* results a good predictor of what will occur *in vivo*. Basically, the methodology employed in most laboratories is closely based on that initially described by Hamburger and Salmon [8, 9]. A brief outline of the basic procedures involved includes:

1. Preparation of single cell suspension – Tumor specimens are received as either pieces of solid tumor in transport media, or malignant effusions or bone marrows to which heparin has been added to prevent clotting. In the case of solid specimens, the tumors are washed with McCoy's 5A media and then minced into small pieces with scissors and passed through a 100-mesh sieve. The cells are then passed through a 25-gauge needle. Liquid specimens are centrifuged and the cell pellet is washed with McCoy's. If large numbers of red cells are present, ammonium chloride lysing buffer is added. In both cases, cell counts are performed in a hemocytometer and a trypan blue estimate of cell viability is made. To ensure good quality of the single cell suspensions, all control plates are examined within the first 24 hours and those with an unacceptable amount of cell clumping are discarded. The production of an adequate single cell suspension in this manner is critical to

the theoretical basis on which the assay is founded, insuring that each colony which is seen is truly a clonal proliferation, arising from one 'stem cell'.

2. Plating the cells in appropriate conditions – The major advance made by the two-layer soft-agar system was its ability to prevent the proliferation of normal fibroblasts. This is accomplished by the simple method of plating the cells on top of an agar underlayer, thus preventing their attachment of fibroblasts to the surface of the plate. Normal fibroblasts are unable to grow without this contact, and thus the system allows for selective tumor cell proliferation.

Basically, the plating of the cells involves the following: the cells to be tested are suspended in 0.3% agar in enriched CMRL-1066 medium supplemented with 15% horse serum, penicillin and streptomycin, glutamine, calcium chloride, and insulin. Just before plating, asparagine, DEAE-dextran, and 2-mercapto-ethanol are added. One milliliter of the solution is then pipetted on top of one-millimeter feeder layers which have been previously prepared in 35-mm plastic petri dishes. The feeder layer consists of McCoy's 5A medium with 15% heat-inactivated fetal calf serum and a variety of nutrients as described by Pike and Robinson [6]. Tryptic soy broth, asparagine, DEAE-dextran, and agar are added immediately before pipetting the solution into the petri dishes. The final concentration of cells on the overlayer is adjusted to 5×10^5 cell/ml before plating. The plates are incubated at 37 °C in a 5% CO_2 humidified atmosphere. Colonies (defined as aggregates of 50 or more cells) are counted on day 14 using an inverted phase microscope.

3. Drug sensitivity testing – The clinical activity of an anti-neoplastic agent involves a number of factors including its ability to inhibit growth of the cells in a particular tumor, its delivery to the tumor, the concentration of the drug in the tumor (which is not always equivalent to the concomitant plasma concentration), the time during which the drug is in contact with the tumor, and the cell cycle kinetics of both the tumor cells and the drug. It is obviously not possible to control all these variables in an *in vitro* system so as to exactly mimic the clinical situation. The kinetics of the tumor cells cannot be easily evaluated nor manipulated, and the vagaries of drug concentration within a solid tumor cannot be duplicated by the single cell suspension used on the stem-cell assay [10]. The two variables which can be easily controlled are the concentration of the drug and the time of the exposure. Although different exposure times including continuous exposure are easily performed, most of the *in vitro/in vivo* correlations to date using this system have been based on one-hour drug exposures. This is therefore the standard in most laboratories. Many drug concentrations have been employed, including ones which are unattainable *in vivo*. In our laboratory we

utilize the somewhat conservative concentration of one-tenth the peak plasma concentration achievable in man. Where a sufficient number of tumor cells are available to permit multiple tests, it is possible to construct dose-response curves by varying the drug concentrations.

Drug sensitivity testing is performed by incubating the single cell suspension with the drug for one hour at 37 °C. Control tubes without drugs are also incubated. After incubation the cells are washed twice to remove the drug, and then suspended in the agar and double-enriched CMRL-1066 media and plated as an overlayer, as described above. All studies are performed in triplicate. The colonies on the plates are counted on day 14 and expressed as a percent reduction in tumor colony-forming units (TCFU's) when compared to control plates (without drug exposure).

2.4. Current problems with the assay

1. Not all tumors grow in the system – Although at least some of the tumors of each histologic type are able to be grown in the system, every patient's tumor does not grow in the assay. Future refinements in media and nutrients utilized and the method of plating may somewhat ameliorate this problem.

2. Low plating efficiency – When 5×10^5 cells per dish are plated, the plating efficiency (number of colonies/number of cells plated) is very low for most tumor types, being usually in the 0.001–0.01 % range. These low values are not unexpected if the stem cell hypothesis is correct. There is, however, a considerable variation between tumor types and among different tumor specimens of the same tumor type. In a specific tumor, the number of colonies formed/cells plated increases to a certain number of cells plated, then actually decreases, probably reflecting media nutrient depletion or waste build-up (see Figure 1). Efforts to increase plating efficiency are con-

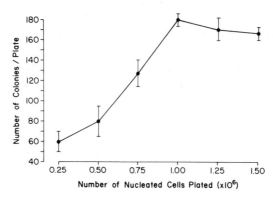

Figure 1. Colonies per plate as a function of number of cells plated in a specimen of squamous cell lung cancer.

tinuously being made. Such an increase would allow for the testing of more anti-neoplastic agents with the same number of tumor cells.

3. Time and expense – The time involved in setting up an assay for a tumor is usually 6–8 hours for solid specimens and somewhat less for effusions. However, a number of tumors can be processed simultaneously with little increase in the time required. The other major time commitment in the past has been that required to count the colonies on each individual plate. This has been circumvented to a large extent by the advent of automatic counters. However, these are expensive and are still in their infancy, requiring at least some confirmation of the validity of the counts on each specimen by visual identification of colonies.

4. Problems with transferring cloning results to clinical decision-making – The major problem in this area is the two-week incubation period to allow for colony growth before drug sensitivity results are available. Attempts are being made to shorten this interval through the use of various radiolabelling techniques instead of colony counting. At the present time, however, these remain of unproven validity. The other major problem involves the determination of drug sensitivity and its correlation with clinical tumor responsiveness. As discussed earlier, the one hour exposure time was an arbitrary choice and may be sub-optimal for some drugs, particularly those that are cell-cycle phase specific agents. The definition of what percent reduction in colonies per plate implies drug sensitivity is also undergoing re-evaluation. A 70% reduction has been used in the past with good *in vitro/in vivo* correlation (see below). However, recent data has suggested that a 50% reduction may be as reliable in at least one tumor type (breast). Others have proposed the necessity for analyzing the results of each tumor separately by using training sets, arriving at a different colony reduction figure for each tumor type.

3. CLONOGENIC ASSAY RESULTS (ALL TUMOR TYPES)

3.1. Demonstration of malignant nature of cells in colonies

One of the questions throughout the development of the clonogenic assay has been whether the cells forming the colonies are in fact tumor cells or whether they could possibly represent growth of normal elements. A number of techniques have been introduced to confirm the presence of tumor cells in different tumor types. Light microscopy of a colony, particularly after it has been made into a histologic slide using a method described by Salmon and Buick [11], can often confirm the neoplastic nature of the cells. Electron microscopy is capable of demonstrating microtubules or desmosomes in tumors of the epithelial origin, confirming the transitional epithelial nature of cells from bladder cancer. Chromosome studies as developed by Trent have demonstrated clonal abnormalities (hypodiploidy and arm deletions) in the cells in colonies from ovarian cancer, bladder cancer, and neuroblastoma [12]. The secretion of tumor markers including somatostatin, melanogens, catecholamines, BETA-HCG, alpha fetoprotein, parathormone, and immunoglobulin, have been demonstrated in a variety of tumors growing in the soft agar system [9, 13, 14], again providing at least circumstantial evidence that the cells are malignant. Nude mouse studies have been done with breast cancer [14] and small cell lung cancer colonies [15]. The production of tumors in these animals again confirms the presence of malignant cells in the colonies.

3.2. Tumor growth

Since the advent of the clonogenic assay, a wide variety of tumors have been grown in the system. The percentage of clinical specimens which produce growth varies from tumor to tumor. Table 1 lists the fraction of each

Table 1. Growth of various tumor histologies in the cloning assay.

Histology	Percent showing growth	
	≥ 5 colonies	≥ 20 colonies
Bladder	49/95 (52)	41/95 (43%)
Brain	56/91 (62%)	45/91 (49%)
Breast	597/1117 (53%)	439/1117 (39%)
Cervix	7/21 (33%)	3/21 (15%)
Colon	192/341 (56%)	148/341 (43%)
Corpus uteri	25/37 (68%)	19/37 (51%)
Esophagus	12/21 (57%)	11/21 (52%)
Kidney	106/150 (71%)	83/150 (55%)
Acute leukemia	17/46 (37%)	9/46 (20%)
Chronic leukemia	3/19 (16%)	2/19 (11%)
Liver	29/44 (66%)	17/44 (37%)
Hodgkin's	30/83 (36%)	16/83 (19%)
Non-hodgkin's lymphoma	82/261 (31%)	42/261 (16%)
Melanoma	76/140 (54%)	63/140 (45%)
Myeloma	18/58 (31%)	10/58 (17%)
Neuroblastoma	77/195 (39%)	51/195 (26%)
Ovary	284/411 (69%)	264/411 (60%)
Pancreas	59/101 (58%)	42/101 (42%)
Prostate	73/142 (51%)	53/142 (37%)
Sarcoma	89/172 (52%)	65/172 (38%)
Stomach	33/70 (47%)	22/70 (29%)
Testis	35/65 (54%)	26/65 (40%)
Thyroid	11/24 (45%)	7/24 (29%)

Table 2. Growth of tumors according to biopsy site.

Source	Percent forming colonies
Malignant effusions	80–90
Bone marrows	80–90
Solid tumors	50–60

individual tumor type producing growth based on the results of over 5000 clinical specimens tested in our laboratory at the University of Texas at San Antonio. As can be seen, multiple tumor histologies are capable of growth in the assay. Higher percentages of some tumor types are capable of producing growth than is true in others. Overall, 50 % of tumors plated result in colony growth with 37 % producing enough colonies (≥ 20) for drug testing.

In addition to the tumor type, an important variable in the ability of a specimen to produce colonies is the source from which the specimen is obtained. When data from a number of tumor types is considered, specimens obtained from bone marrows and malignant effusions produce growth more often than do solid specimens (Table 2).

A more detailed description of the data for the various histologic types of lung cancer will be presented later in this chapter.

3.3. In vitro/in vivo correlations of drug sensitivity testing results

The major clinical application of the stem-cell assay system is its use in attempting to predict the response of a patient's tumor *in vivo* based on the results of *in vitro* drug testing. The initial report of the possibility of such a correlation was made by Salmon and his colleagues [16]. They tested the tumors from 18 patients with either ovarian cancer or multiple myeloma in the stem cell assay in either a prospective or retrospective manner. These patients were treated with one of the drugs which were tested *in vitro* and a comparison was made between the sensitivity or resistance to the drug as determined *in vitro* and the clinical response of the patient's tumor. Of the eleven cases where the tumor was sensitive *in vitro*, 10/11 showed clinical sensitivity. Of the twenty instances of *in vitro* resistance, clinical resistance was seen in all twenty.

Because of this data in this small group of patients, a large retrospective analysis was conducted by Von Hoff and associates [17]. Out of a total of 800 specimens, 123 fulfilled the criteria for an *in vitro/in vivo* correlation; namely, the tumor produced enough colonies in the assay to allow for drug testing and the patient was treated with at least one of the drugs tested. The tumors included multiple histologies, and both standard and experimental drugs were tested. There were 21 instances in which the assay predicted that the drug would be effective. Clinical response was seen in 15/21 (70%) of these cases. When the assay predicted resistance to the drug, clinical response was only seen in 2/100 (2%). Thus, this study confirms the strong predictive value of the results of the clonogenic assay in determining patients response to individual neoplastic agents. In particular, lack of sensitivity in the assay to a particular drug makes it quite unlikely (2% of cases) that the patient's tumor would respond to that drug clinically. One problem identified by the authors is the low rate of identifying a clinically active drug (15/800 specimens). The major reason for this was the fact that only 25% of the specimens produced enough colonies for drug sensitivity testing and of these, only about 60% of the patients were treated with one of the drugs tested. The significant percentage of false positives (30%) among those agents identified as active is disturbing. As discussed previously, these could be due to problems with the assay technique and definitions (one hour drug exposure, drug concentration used, definition of sensitivity) or could be due to variables in the patient (poor delivery of drug to the tumor, possible antagonism between drugs used in combination). An additional point raised by the authors is the possibility that the assay is not valuable so much in selecting a particular drug which will be active but rather in selecting tumors which are responsive to standard chemotherapeutic agents in general.

Despite the problems discussed above, current evidence suggests strongly that the clonogenic assay can be a good predictor of clinical response. This is particularly true in a negative sense (lack of response in the assay predicting clinical resistance) and has the potential of saving many patients from the toxicities of these drugs. Further data is clearly needed and a prospective trial of single agent chemotherapy correlated with assay results is currently being done and will hopefully answer many of the remaining questions. Further studies are planned to compare treatment based on assay results *versus* empiric drug selection by the clinician to determine if drug selection by the assay can truly provide benefit to the patient.

4. THE CLONOGENIC ASSAY IN LUNG CANCER

The potential usefulness of the stem-cell assay in the management of lung cancer patients is a topic of considerable interest because of the generally dismal results of current management of this group of diseases. For each of the histologic subtypes, information will be presented as to the ability to grow the tumor in the assay and the results of drug sensitivity testing with a variety of agents. Because responses to anti-neoplastic agents are much more common with small cell cancer than with the other histologies, more detailed information will be given on this subtype, including possible application of the assay for diagnosis, prognosis, staging, and screening for new active agents.

4.1. Small cell cancer

1. Diagnosis – The cloning assay has potential for improving the diagnostic yield from bronchoscopy in patients with small cell lung cancer. In this regard, Von Hoff and associates attempted to clone the cells obtained from bronchial washings and to correlate the presence or absence of growth with the cytology [18]. Of the 7 patients with cytologies positive for small cell carcinoma, 5/7 (72%) produced growth in the assay. However, utilizing the presently accepted criteria of 5 colonies per plate as a definition of growth, only 2/7 (28%) of these would be considered positive for growth. Again using this definition, 8/8 cytologically negative specimens showed no growth in the assay (2 specimens produced 1 and 3 colonies, respectively). Of additional interest is the fact that 4/4 of the non-small cell lung cancers with positive cytology demonstrated growth in the assay. Thus, the stem-cell assay is able to show growth in bronchscopically obtained bronchial washings in patients with lung cancer. Whether it will produce diagnostic information beyond that provided by routine studies (that is, positive assay growth demonstrating the presence of tumor despite no tumor being detectable by visual inspection, biopsies, and cytologies from the bronchial tree) will require further studies.

Of perhaps more interest regarding the question of whether the assay can provide information to and in the diagnosis and staging of small cell lung cancer is the data presented by our group at the Stem Cell Conference in Tucson, in January 1982 [19]. Out of a group of 165 specimens obtained from patients with biopsy proven small cell lung cancer, 99 of the specimens were negative for tumor at the time of routine pathologic examination (es-

Table 3. Concordance of assay growth and pathology results in bone marrows from patients with small cell carcinoma.

Assay	Pathology	
	Positive	Negative
Positive	6	11
Negative	9	69

Concordance: 75/95 (72%)

Table 4. Concordance of assay growth and pathology results in effusions from patients with small cell carcinoma.

	Pathology	
	Positive	Negative
Positive	10	2
Negative	2	15

Concordance: 25/29 (86%)

sentially all representing bone marrow examinations done for staging (80) and effusions (17)). Despite the negative pathology on part of the same specimen, 14% of the bone marrows and 11% of the effusions nonetheless produced growth in the assay ($\geqslant 5$ colonies per plate) (Tables 3 and 4). Most of the colonies were no longer available for further analysis, but in 2 specimens, nude mouse studies and electron micrographs confirmed the malignant nature of the cells [15].

Because of the question as to whether the assay results represented false positive findings or whether the pathology was falsely negative, an analysis was made of survival of subset of this group of patients who had their specimens submitted at the time of the initial diagnosis. The question to be answered was whether their survival approximated that of other patients with limited or extensive disease. The hypothesis that was advanced was that if the assay positivity truly reflected the presence of malignant calls in the bone marrow, the survival of the patients should approximate that of other patients with extensive disease. If, however, the assay was falsely positive and the patients did not in fact have malignant cells in these biopsy sites (as predicted by routine pathology), then their survival should be close to that of other patients with limited disease. The survival curves for patients with limited and extensive disease as well as that of the subjects with the assay-positive, histology-negative phenomenon are shown in Figure 2.

Because of the very small number of subjects in the test group, statistically significant differences were unlikely. Upon evaluation, the survival of the assay-positive, pathology-negative patients could not be differentiated from either patients with limited or extensive disease. However, at the time of follow-up, the actual percent survival in this group of patients had fallen below that of patients with extensive disease. This suggests that, with more patients and longer follow-up, these patients could be shown to behave as if they had extensive disease. If this is in fact the case, it would indicate that

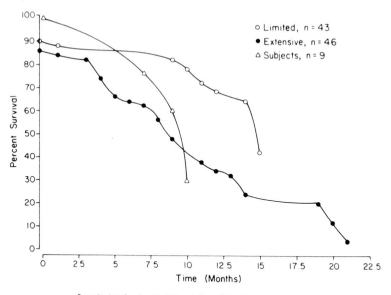

Figure 2. Survival curve for assay-positive, histology-negative patients with small cell lung cancer compared to survival curves of other patients with limited or extensive disease.

the clonogenic assay is capable of detecting metastatic disease in a significant number of bone marrow and effusion specimens (13%) which are thought to be negative on routine pathologic examination. If this proves to be true, the human tumor cloning assay would conceivably become part of the staging work-up in patients with small cell lung cancer.

2. Growth in the assay – Of the 66 histologically positive small cell lung cancer specimens in the study described above, 43/66 (64%) produced growth in the assay. Thirty-three of the 66 (50%) produced at least 30 colonies per control plate, allowing for meaningful drug testing results. When growth rates were analyzed as to specimen source, the following

Table 5. Growth of small cell carcinoma according to specimen source.

Specimen source	Percent with growth	
Bone marrow	6/15	(40%)
Solid tumors	27/39	(69%)
Malignant effusions	10/12	(83%)
Total	43/66	(64%)

Table 6. Growth of small cell carcinoma based on previous therapy.

Category	Percent with growth
Previous therapy	12/21 (57%)
No previous therapy	32/46 (69%)

Groups not statistically different.

emerged: malignant effusions grew very well with 83% producing assay growth. Solid tumor specimens had intermediate growth potential with a rate of 69%. Bone marrows (unlike the previously described results in all tumor types) showed the lowest fraction of specimens demonstrating growth (40%), possibly related to low numbers of tumor stem cells in the specimens (Table 5).

The ability of the specimens to grow in the assay was also analyzed on the basis of whether or not the patient had received previous chemotherapy. The results with (12/21 = 57%) and without (32/46 = 69%) prior therapy were not significantly different (Table 6).

3. Drug sensitivity testing – The results of drug sensitivity testing in specimens containing small cell carcinoma of the lung are shown in Table 7. Results are displayed for a 50% reduction in tumor colony-forming units. Only those agents which were utilized in at least 5 drug tests are displayed.

Inspection of the data reveals a number of interesting points. The clinical activity of many of the standard drugs in the treatment of this disease (e.g. adriamycin, vincristine, and methotrexate) is confirmed by the finding that a significant number of tumor specimens are also sensitive to these drugs *in vitro*. The only exception to this is VP-16 which is a very active drug in the clinical setting but which inhibited growth in only a small percentage of

Table 7. Drug sensitivity results for small cell carcinoma.

Drug	Percent with at least 50% reduction in tumor colony-forming units
Vincristine	6/14 (43%)
Methotrexate	3/10 (30%)
VP-16	2/12 (16%)
Adriamycin	7/20 (35%)
Mitoxantrone	4/14 (29%)
Bisantrene	7/11 (64%)
Chlorambucil	2/12 (16%)
Cis-platinum	3/6 (50%)

tumors *in vitro*. This discrepancy is thought to be due to difficulties with suspension of the drug in the vehicle used in the assay.

The second aspect to be considered is a comparison of adriamycin and the new anthracene derivative drugs Bisantrene (anthracenedicarboxalde-hyde) and Mitoxantrone (dihydroxyanthracenedione, DHAD). Of these three drugs, Bisantrene demonstrates the highest rate of activity in the assay. This holds true even when the results are controlled for previous adriamycin therapy. This suggests that Bisantrene could be a very active clinical drug in small cell cancer, and a Phase II trial is currently underway to evaluate this possibility. In addition, because of the presence of some (albeit small) activity *in vitro*, a trial of Mitoxantrone would be of interest. Such a trial has recently been completed in the Southwest Oncology Group with 0/35 patients with disease refractory to previous chemotherapy showing any objective response. In 14 other patients without previous adriamycin therapy, 2/14 had an objective response [20].

The third point which should be considered in evaluating *in vitro* drug results is the possibility of detecting a drug which might possess clinical activity which had not been previously recognized (drug screening function). Such a drug in small cell cancer could be Cis-platinum. As can be seen, in a

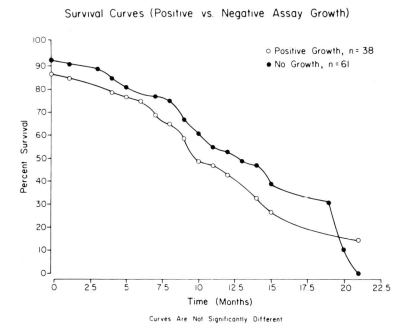

Figure 3. Survival curves for patients with small cell lung cancer grouped by the presence or absence of tumor growth in the clonogenic assay (all patients).

64

small number of trials (6), it appeared to possess significant activity (50%
response rate). Although it has not been shown to have high clinical activity
in early clinical trials [21], when combined with other agents, high response
rates have been noted [22, 23].

Thus, drug sensitivity testing in specimens of small cell lung cancer seems
to perform three functions. It confirms the activity of many of the standard
agents (and conceivably could predict which should be used in a single
patient), it allows for a comparison of drugs which resemble each other in
structure and function, and it functions as a screening test for potentially
active drugs.

4. Prognostic implications – The final point to consider is whether presence of growth in the assay could conceivably be a prognostically important factor. This has been done in our patiens through the means of con-
structing survival curves for those patients with and without growth in the
assay. When these curves are examined in all patients (Figure 3) and in the
subset of patients with extensive disease, there is no difference between the
two curves. However, when only those patients with limited disease are
included (Figure 4), the curves are statistically significant different, with
those patients whose tumors produced growth in the assay having a worse
prognosis.

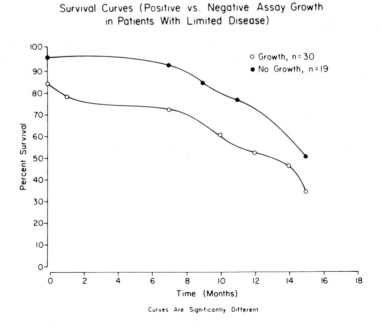

Figure 4. Survival curves for patients with small cell lung cancer grouped by the presence or
absence of tumor growth in the clonogenic assay (patients with limited disease only).

The exact explanation for these findings is at present unknown. On hypothesis would be that these tumors which grew in the assay would be inherently biologically more aggressive, with a tendency to metastasize earlier. This factor would not be important in those patients who already had extensive (metastatic) disease, but in those patients without metastases (the limited group), it could select out those prone to develop earlier dissemination and thus having a worse prognosis. Whether this hypothesis is confirmed or refuted will only become obvious with the advent of more sophisticated methodologies for determining biologic aggressiveness and metastatic potential. For the present, however, one is able to conclude that the ability of a tumor to grow in the stem-cell assay does have prognostic import for those patients with clinically limited disease.

5. OTHER LUNG CANCER HISTOLOGIES (NON-SMALL CELL)

1. Growth in the assay – As can be appreciated from Table 8, the precent of specimens from patients with non-small cell cancer which produce growth in the assay is comparable to that seen with small cell cancer (61% versus 64%). However, significantly fewer specimens are capable of producing enough growth (≥30 colonies per plate) to allow for drug sensitivity testing (37% versus 50% for small cell). Among the individual histologies, the most likely one to produce growth is large cell carcinoma (72%) followed by adenocarcinoma (67%) and squamous cell (57%). A similar trend is seen for tumors producing enough colonies for drug testing with large cell cancer growing in a frequency (48%) essentially equal to that seen in small cell carcinoma. One factor which may make this growth potential appear poorer than it actually is is the fact that, unlike in the small cell tumors, we have not completed verification of the pathology in all the specimens received. This should be a minor problem at most, however, since sampling

Table 8. Growth of non-oat cell lung cancer.

Histology	Percent of specimens producing growth			
	≥ 5 colonies		≥ 30 colonies	
Adenocarcinoma	96/156	(62%)	60/156	(38%)
Squamous cell	75/133	(57%)	40/133	(31%)
Large cell	36/50	(72%)	24/50	(48%)
Total (non-oat cell)	207/339	(61%)	124/339	(37%)
Total (including oat cell)	250/405	(62%)	157/405	(39%)

Table 9. Growth of non-small cell lung cancer by biopsy site.

| | Percent of specimens with growth (≥ 5 colonies) | | | |
| | Biopsy site | | | |
Histology	Pleura (effusions and biopsies)	Bone marrow	Solid tumor[a]	Other[b]
Adenocarcinoma	33/62 (53%)	3/11 (27%)	54/77 (70%)	6/8 (75%)
Squamous cell	15/33 (45%)	1/5 (20%)	52/85 (61%)	4/9 (44%)
Large cell	6/10 (60%)	4/5 (80%)	26/33 (79%)	0/2 (0%)
Total	54/105 (51%)	8/21 (38%)	132/195 (68%)	10/19 (53%)

[a] 'Solid tumor' category includes primary tumors and solid metastases.
[b] 'Other' category includes ascites fluid, and CSF.
No attempt was made to verify whether the pathologic examinations were positive or negative for tumor.

procedures without evidence of disease (i.e. bone marrows) are done much less frequently in these diseases.

2. Growth according to tissue source – The data for growth according to specimen source is presented in Table 9 for each of the histologies. Among both solid tumors (primary lesions and solid metastases) and pleural disease (effusions and direct extension of tumor), the same patterns of growth are seen; namely, large cell carcinoma being the most likely to produce growth followed by adenocarcinoma and squamous cell, in that order. Solid tumors grew significantly more often than did pleural disease (68% *versus* 51%) but this is again subject to the qualification that pleural disease, particularly effusions, are much more likely to be negative for tumor cells than are solid tumor deposits. The data for bone marrows and 'other' metastases (usually ascitic fluid or CSF) are too scanty to allow for any meaningful conclusions.

3. Drug sensitivity testing – A large number of standard and experimental anti-neoplastic agents were tested against specimens of the various lung cancer histologies. The results are shown in Table 10 for all drugs that were tested against at least 5 specimens of a given histology. As a general statement, it can easily be seen that few drugs appear to have activity against a significant percentage of the tumors of any histology. Exceptions to this rule appear to be two of the drugs tested against large cell carcinoma: vinblastine (activity seen in 5/5 trials) and Bisantrene (activity in 3/8 trials). This positive data suggests the possible value of future clinical trials of these agents in patients with large cell cancer. This general lack of *in vitro* activity is not surprising, given the resistant nature of these tumors *in vivo*. Somewhat

Table 10. Drug sensitivity testing results[a] for non-small cell lung cancer.

Drug	Percent decrease in tumor colony-forming units (TCFUs)					
	Adeno		Large cell		Squamous	
	≥70%	≥50%	≥70%	≥50%	≥70%	≥50%
5-FU	0/24 (0%)	1/24 (4%)	0/6 (0%)	1/6 (17%)	0/10 (0%)	1/10 (10%)
Adriamycin	0/52 (0%)	5/52 (10%)	0/13 (0%)	1/13 (7%)	1/22 (5%)	2/22 (19%)
Bisantrene	2/22 (96%)	4/22 (18%)	3/8 (37%)	4/8 (50%)	2/16 (12%)	4/16 (25%)
Chlorambucil	1/32 (3%)	4/32 (12%)	0/10 (0%)	0/10 (0%)	1/21 (5%)	4/19 (19%)
DHAD	1/30 (3%)	3/30 (10%)	1/10 (10%)	3/10 (30%)	4/19 (21%)	6/19 (32%)
Mitomycin-C	1/17 (6%)	2/17 (12%)	0/6 (0%)	0/6 (0%)	2/10 (20%)	3/10 (30%)
Cis-platinum	0/26 (0%)	2/26 (8%)	1/10 (10%)	4/10 (40%)	1/17 (6%)	4/17 (23%)
Vincristine	0/19 (0%)	3/19 (16%)	1/5 (20%)	2/5 (40%)	2/8 (25%)	3/8 (37%)
Vinblastine	2/14 (14%)	3/14 (21%)	5/5 (100%)	5/5 (100%)	–	–
M-ASMA	0/7 (0%)	2/7 (29%)	–	–	–	–
MGBG	1/6 (17%)	1/6 (17%)	1/6 (17%)	2/6 (33%)	0/13 (0%)	0/13 (0%)
Bleomycin	–	–	–	–	1/7 (14%)	1/7 (14%)
Methotrexate	2/11 (18%)	2/11 (18%)	–	–	–	–
Interferon	1/5 (20%)	1/5 (20%)	–	–	–	–

[a] For drugs tested against at least 5 tumor specimens.

disturbing, however, is the lack of *in vitro* activity for some of the agents which have shown some *in vivo* activity (e.g. 5-FU, vincristine, and mito-mycin-C(FOMi) in adenocarcinoma and large cell carcinoma). This apparent lack of correlation may be due to any one of a number of factors including insufficient data, synergism *in vivo* with the drug combination, or previous treatment with anti-neoplastic drugs leading to less *in vitro* sensitivity. A definitive answer to this question will only be obtained when *in vitro* and *in vivo* testing are compared in the same patient group in a prospective manner.

An additional point to be considered in evaluating the drug sensitivity data is the question posed previously; namely, does activity of one or more drugs simply select out a chemosensitive group of tumors rather than suggesting a specific agent for an individual tumor. The data does not allow a definitive answer to this question, but it is interesting to consider the overall sensitivity rates in the individual histologic subtypes. Of all the drug tests done in large cell carcinoma, a reduction of $\geqslant 70\%$ in tumor colony-forming units (TCFUs) was seen in 15%. Similar figures for squamous cell carcinoma and adenocarcinoma were 10% and 4%, respectively. It is unclear at the present whether these differences represent differences in the biologic nature of the various tumor types or whether they are in large part a function of the drugs which are selected for testing.

Thus, it has been shown that non-oat cell cancers can be grown in the stem-cell system and drug sensitivity testing can be performed in over a third of the specimens submitted. Rates of drug activity in these tumors are generally much lower than those seen in small cell carcinoma, corresponding to the clinically-recognized increased resistance of these tumor types. No new agents for clinical trials are suggested by the data presented other than perhaps vinblastine and Bisantrene for large cell carcinoma. Data on the usefulness of the assay in prognosis and staging like that presented for small cell carcinoma, is not presently available. Similarly, detailed prospective *in vitro/in vivo* correlations have not yet been accomplished for these tumors.

6. CONCLUSIONS

The soft-agar clonogenic system is based on the stem-cell hypothesis. This states that a certain small percentage of cells in a given tumor are capable of reproducing themselves and also giving rise to a large number of more differentiated progeny. It is these cells which, when put in the soft-agar system, are each presumably capable to giving rise to a colony of malignant cells, composed of one clone. Continuous refinements have allowed achievement of the present situation wherein one-half of all tumor specimens of varying histologic types received have produced growth in the assay system. There are still a number of problems with the system including the fact that one-half of tumors fail to produce growth, the time and expense involved in performing the assay itself, and the low plating efficiency even when growth is achieved.

Once a tumor produces growth in the assay, the results of drug sensitivity testing can be evaluated. Problems include the limited number of drugs which can be tested against an individual tumor (a function of the low plating efficiency mentioned above), and the two-week delay before results are available to the clinician. Initial evaluations of correlations between *in vitro* results of drug testing and *in vivo* tumor response have been most encouraging for the use of the system as a predictor of clinical drug activity (and even more encouraging for predicting drug resistance).

Extensive data accumulation for specimens from patients with small cell lung cancer has shown that the tumors are capable of growth in almost two-thirds of cases and drug sensitivity testing can be done in half of the specimens submitted. Malignant effusions and metastatic disease grow the best, with bone marrow specimens being the worst. Primary tumors and lymph node metastases occupy an intermediate position. Previous chemotherapy has no effect on growth potential. Drug testing results confirm the activity of standard clinically-utilized agents and suggest possible new drugs for clinical trials (Cis-platinum, Bisantrene). In addition, growth in the assay is a negative prognostic factor for patients with clinically limited disease. The assay may also eventually be utilized in staging patients because of its potential ability to detect metastases in bone marrows and effusions which may be missed on routine pathology. This latter point must be regarded as conjectural at the present time, however, pending more data.

The data available for non-small cell lung cancers contains a large number of clinical specimens, but detailed analyses of patient characteristics and follow-up are not yet available as they are for small cell carcinoma. These tumors can be grown in the assay and drug sensitivity testing done (although less often than in small cell carcinoma). Large cell carcinoma produces growth most often and squamous cell least often. Drugs tested against these tumors seldom show activity against a high percentage of specimens.

Future goals are for manipulations of the system to allow for a greater growth of tumors and the ability to test more drugs through increased plating efficiency. Further well-done prospective *in vitro/in vivo* testing is necessary before the assay can be seen as having a role in the routine management of patients with malignancy.

ACKNOWLEDGMENT

This work was supported in part by Medical Oncology Program Project Grant No. CA30195.

REFERENCES

1. Von Hoff DD, Wiesenthal L: *In vitro* methods to predict for patient response to chemotherapy. Adv in Pharm and Chemother 17:133–156, 1980.
2. Von Hoff DD, Harris GJ, Johnson G, Glaubiger D: Initial experience with the human tumor stem cell assay system: Potential and problems. In: Cloning of Human Tumor Stem Cells. Salmon SE (ed). New York: Liss, 1980, pp 113–124.
3. Von Hoff DD: A human tumor stem cell system: Concepts, methodology, and application. In: Cancer and Chemotherapy III. Crooke ST and Prestayko AW (eds). Academic Press, 1981, pp 207–218.
4. Salmon SE, Von Hoff DD: *In vitro* evaluation of anti-cancer drugs with the human tumor stem cell assay. Sem in Oncol 8:377–385, 1981.
5. Steel GC: Cell kinetics and cell survival. In: Medical Oncology – Medical Aspects of Malignant Disease. Bagshane KD (ed). Oxford: Blackwell Scientific Publication, 1975, pp 49–66.
6. Pike BL, Robinson WA: Human bone marrow colony growth in agar-gel. J Cell Physiol 76:77–84, 1970.
7. Bruce WR, Meeker BE, Baleriote FA: Comparison of the sensitivity of normal hematopoietic and transplanted lymphoma colony-forming cells to chemotherapeutic agents administered *in vivo*. J Natl Cancer Inst 37:233–245, 1966.
8. Hamburger AW, Salmon SE: Primary bioassay of human tumor stem cells. Science 197:461–463, 1977.
9. Hamburger AW, Salmon SE: Primary bioassay of human myeloma stem cells. J Clin Invest 60:846–854, 1977.
10. Cline MJ: *In vitro* test systems for anti-cancer drugs. NEJM 280:955, 1969 (editorial).
11. Salmon SE, Buick RM: Preparation of permanent slides of intact soft agar colony cultures of hematopoietic and tumor stem cells. Cancer Res 39–1133–1136, 1979.
12. Trent JM: Cytogenetic analysis of human tumor cells cloned in agar. In: Cloning of Human Tumor Stem Cells. Salmon SE (ed). New York: Liss, 1980, pp 165–177.
13. Von Hoff DD, Johnson GE: Secretion of tumor markers in the human tumor stem cell assay system. Proc Am Assoc Cancer Res 20–51, 1979 (abstract).
14. Von Hoff DD: New leads from the laboratory for treating testicular cancer. In: Proc of Recent Advances in the Treatment of Ovarian and Testicular Cancer. Noordwijkerhout, The Netherlands, Dec. 6–8, 1979, pp 81–82.
15. Pollard EB, Tio F, Myers JW, Clark G, Coltman CA Jr, Von Hoff DD: Utilization of a human tumor cloning system to monitor for marrow involvement with small cell carcinoma of the lung. Cancer Res 41:1015–1020, 1981.
16. Salmon SE, Hamburger AW, Soehnlen B, Durie BGM, Alberts DS, Moon TE: Quantitation of differential sensitivity of human-tumor stem cells to anticancer drugs. NEJM 298:1321–1327, 1978.
17. Von Hoff DD, Casper J, Bradley E, Sandbach J, Jones D and Makuch R: Association between human tumor colony-forming assay results and response of an individual patient's tumor to chemotherapy. Am J Med 70:1027–1032, 1981.

18. Von Hoff DD, Wiesenthal LM, Ihde DC, Mathews MJ, Layard M, Makuch R: Growth in lung cancer colonies from bronchoscopy washings. Cancer 48:400–403, 1981.
19. Callahan SK, Von Hoff DD: Growth of oat cell carcinoma of the lung in the human tumor cloning assay. Third Conference on Human Tumor Cloning, January 10–12, 1982, Tucson, Az., p 28 (abstract).
20. Von Hoff DD, Clark GM, Callahan SK, Livingston R: Southwest Oncology Group Trial of mitoxantrone in patients with refractory small cell cancer of the lung. Cancer Treat Rep (in press).
21. Dombernowsky P, Sorensen J, Aisner J, Hansen HH: Cis-dichlorodiammineplatinum (II) in small cell anaplastic bronchogenic carcinoma: A Phase II study. Cancer Treat Rep 63:543–545, 1979.
22. Sierocki JS, Hicaris BS, Hopfan S, Martini N, Breton D, Golbey RB, Wittes RE: Cis-dichlorodiammineplatinum (II) and VP-16-213: An active induction regimen for small cell cancer of the lung. Cancer Treat Rep 63: 1593-1597, 1979.
23. Eagen RT, Frytak S, Nichols WC, Ingle JN, Creagen CT, Kvois LK: Cyclophosphamide and VP-16-213 with or without Cisplatin in squamous cell and small cell lung cancers. Cancer Treat Rep 65:453–458, 1981.

5. Autologous Bone Marrow Transplantation – Potential Usefulness in Lung Cancer Management

STEVEN N. WOLFF

1. INTRODUCTION

The therapeutic use of bone marrow transplantation (BMTX) has proliferated in the past few years. Once considered a desperate attempt to control end-stage refractory leukemia, BMTX is now used to treat acute leukemia in remission [1, 2], chronic myelogenous leukemia [3], non-Hodgkin's lymphoma [4], some solid tumors [5], aplastic anemia [6], and the malignant process osteopetrosis [7]. Initially limited to histocompatible siblings (allogeneic transplantation) or monozygotic twins (syngeneic transplantation), the ability to cryopreserve marrow for prolonged periods fostered autologous bone marrow transplantation (ABMTX) in which the patient serves as both marrow donor and recipient. In addition to removing histocompatibility restraints, ABMTX eliminates the requirement for pre-transplant immunosuppression to prevent graft rejection and lessens the potential of graft-*vs*-host disease [8].

Although only a few studies using ABMTX in lung cancer have been undertaken, the increasing use of this technique makes this review timely. This chapter will focus on the concepts and techniques of ABMTX and review some of the ongoing studies in lung cancer.

2. RATIONALE OF HIGH-DOSE THERAPY WITH ABMTX

Standard cytotoxic therapy, whether single agent or combination of agents is constructed to be tumoricidal and 'tolerable' with respect to normal tissue toxicity. Dose and schedule of drug administration is titrated to achieve that balance. Organs with rapid cellular proliferation rates such as the bone marrow and intestinal mucosa are commonly adversely affected by and limit cytotoxic therapy. Although modest degrees of cytotoxic therapy

Greco, FA (ed), Biology and Management of Lung Cancer. ISBN 0-89838-554-7.
© *1983, Martinus Nijhoff Publishers, Boston. Printed in The Netherlands.*

induced bone marrow suppression can be tolerated by most patients, profound disturbances resulting in severe neutropenia and thrombocytopenia can be devastating [9, 10]. Presumably, the rapid recovery of normal tissue compared to neoplastic tissue allows for cumulative tumor toxicity with repeated courses of therapy [11]. Bone marrow recovery generally limits the intensity and frequency of cytotoxic therapy.

Chemotherapy and radiation therapy like many other pharmacologic interventions demonstrate dose-response relationships in *in vitro* systems, animal models and in some human tumors [12]. Dose-response relationships become meaningful when a high dose capable of killing most or all of the tumor cannot be given because of host toxicity. Dose-response relationships become particularly meaningful when the curve is steep realizing significant increments in tumor cytotoxicity with increasing dose as opposed to flat curves in which only modest increments in cytotoxicity occur.

Ionizing radiation, alkylating agents and the nitrosoureas have demonstrated steep dose-response relationships [13]. Hodgkin's disease control by ionizing radiation has been well studied and demonstrates a steep dose-response relationship [14]. At 1000 rads, the tumor recurrence rate is 60%, decreasing to 35% at 2000 rads, 18% at 3000 rads and less than 10% at 4000–4500 rads. Using various chemotherapeutic agents, there are now provocative examples of *in vitro* and animal data which have been applied to human studies. For example, melphalan, an alkylating agent demonstrates a steep dose-response curve in the murine B16 melanoma [15]. Against human melanoma, melphalan at standard dose has a response rate of 15% [16]. Using high-dose melphalan followed by ABMTX, response rates of over 50% have been achieved with some complete regressions noted [17]. In a similar fashion, the nitrosourea BCNU demonstrates a steep dose-response curve *in vitro* [18]. When used against human melanoma in clinical trial, BCNU has demonstrated a marked increase in response rate with high-dose therapy [19].

In my laboratory, *in vitro* observations of a steep dose-response curve have been demonstrated with the epipodophylotoxin, VP16-213. Standard clinical doses of VP16-213 produce plasma levels of less than 20 µg/ml [20]. In a variety of murine tumors in suspension culture complete cytotoxicity with brief drug exposure requires VP16-213 levels of 20 µg/ml or more [21]. Applying this *in vitro* information to patients, VP16-213 was escalated using a modified Fibonacci scheme in a high-dose Phase I trial. Peak plasma levels achieved with the higher doses exceeded that required for complete cytotoxicity in the *in vitro* models. Patients with extensive small cell carcinoma of the lung have been given high-dose VP16-213 and preliminary results reveal a response rate higher than that reported with standard doses [22].

In addition to single agent studies, some refractory patients with leukemia, lymphoma and germ cell tumors have been cured by high-dose therapy and this also supports the concept of high-dose therapy. However, limitations exist for dose-response relationships since not all chemotherapeutic agents exhibit steep dose-response curves, and many drugs cannot be used at above standard doses due to prohibitive toxicities [23]. In addition, absolute dose may not be the sole determinant of cytotoxicity since both duration of drug exposure and frequency of exposure can be important factors [24].

Assuming the clinical value of steep dose-response relationships, ABMTX provides a mechanism of administering high-dose therapy when the dose-limiting toxicity is bone marrow suppression. Much higher doses of therapy could be given and the patient's bone marrow would be reconstituted by the transplant. ABMTX is required to guarantee restoration of hematopoiesis if the high-dose therapy is marrow ablative. ABMTX may also be justified if the high-dose therapy produces a prolonged duration of severe cytopenias. In addition, ABMTX may also be useful to replace a pool of damaged stem cells when cytotoxic therapy produces cumulative as opposed to acute marrow toxicity.

3. TECHNIQUES OF ABMTX

ABMTX was first presented in the medical literature in the 1950s but did not become clinically useful until more effective chemotherapy and patient support techniques became available. At present ABMTX is performed at many major medical centers and the number of institutions is rapidly increasing. Although variations of techniques exist for harvest, cryopreservation and reinfusion, a standard method used at Vanderbilt University and by other institutions in the Southeastern Cancer Study Group is summarized in Table 1.

3.1. Marrow harvest

Before harvest, a diagnostic marrow examination (aspiration and biopsy) is performed to assess cellularity and whether there is evidence of metastatic tumor. Normal marrow (greater than 40% cellular) associated with normal peripheral blood counts is considered suitable. Although augmentation of marrow progenitor cells shortly after chemotherapy has been described, we prefer not to collect marrow with recent chemotherapy [25]. The marrow donor is placed in the prone position under general or regional anesthesia. Using sterile technique large bone marrow needles are inserted simultaneously in both posterior iliac crests by two operators. Approximately 5 to

Table 1. Techniques of ABMTX.

1. Determine adequacy of marrow status
2. Harvest by multiple percutaneous aspirations from posterior iliac crest under regional or general anesthesia
3. Anticoagulate with heparin (10 units/ml) and continually mix the collected marrow
4. Remove large debris and make a single cell suspension by sequential filtering thru stainless steel mesh (0.3 and 0.2 mm)
5. Place in standard blood bag for transport
6. Deplete 80% of plasma by centrifugation (4000 RPM × 10 min at 22 °C)
7. Prepare buffy coat by centrifugation in siliconized glass test tubes (2500 RPM × 15 min at 22 °C)
8. Separate and pool buffy coat by needle aspiration
9. Mix with freezing solution yielding a final concentration of 10% DMSO and 20% autologous plasma
10. Freeze in a programmable freezer at 1 °C/min from 0 to −80 °C
11. Store in liquid nitrogen
12. Administer by rapid thawing in a 37 °C water bath and reinfuse intravenously immediately over 5 minutes

10 ml of marrow are then aspirated. The needles are inserted further into the crests with aspiration approximately every one cm. Care is taken not to aspirate large quantities of marrow from each location and as much of the posterior crest as possible is aspirated. Immediately after aspiration, the marrow is anticoagulated with heparin (10 units/ml) and continually mixed. With proper technique, the total volume of marrow required for satisfactory cell quantity is approximately 10 ml/kg representing less than 5% of the total body marrow pool. Marrow donation is well tolerated with postoperative pain at the sites of aspiration as the major complication. Since peripheral blood is aspirated along with the marrow some patients may require red blood cell transfusions during harvest since approximately 15% of blood volume may be collected with the marrow. If intraoperative transfusions are required the blood must be irradiated to greater than 1500 rads to eliminate the collection and possible reinfusion with the marrow of viable allogeneic cells which could cause graft-*vs*-host disease. For patients with normal hematocrits able to donate blood, autologous red blood cell transfusion after liquid storage adequately replaces blood lost during harvest.

3.2. Marrow processing

Although some investigators cryopreserve and transplant unseparated marrow, the large volume of plasma, red blood cells, fat and mature leucocytes encouraged separation of these elements [26]. After anticoagulation and mixing, the marrow is passed thru stainless steel mesh (0.3 and 0.2 mm) to remove gross particulate matter and evenly suspend the cells. The marrow is next placed in plastic bags for centrifugation. Using standard blood banking techniques, the marrow is centrifuged to remove 80% of the plasma. The packed marrow is then mixed, placed in siliconized glass test tubes and centrifuged (2500 RPM × 15 min at 22°C) to form a distinct buffy coat. By aspirating the buffy coat most of the remaining plasma, fat and red blood cells can be eliminated. From an initial volume of 700 ml, approximately 70 ml of buffy coat material is separated for cryopreservation. In addition to this technique, marrow cells may be separated and collected by Ficoll-Hypaque gradients and collection of the mononuclear interface or by using an automated intermittent flow cell separator such as the Haemonetics model 30 to process the harvested marrow. The latter two techniques are technically more demanding, cumbersome, time-consuming and expensive.

3.3. Cryopreservation

The theory of cryopreservation and the prevention of freeze injury are described in detail in a recent review [27]. Basic requirements for marrow preservation are generally accepted as: (1) the marrow be frozen at a linear rate of 1–3°C/min from 0 to −80°C; (2) a cryoprotective agent such as dimethyl sulfoxide (DMSO) (final concentration 10%) be used; (3) since 10% DMSO is toxic to cells at warm temperatures, the interval of time once DMSO is added to the cells before freezing must be minimized; (4) the heat generated by the transition from liquid to solid be abrogated as quickly as possible; (5) the final plasma concentration be at least 20%. These requirements are achieved using a programmable freezer cooled by bursts of liquid nitrogen. In our laboratory the marrow suspension is mixed 1:1 with a freezing solution (20% DMSO, 40% autologous plasma, 40% tissue culture media) and placed in polyolefin plastic freezing bags resulting in the appropriate freezing concentrations. The bags, each containing 100 ml of marrow are compressed between aluminium plates (maximum thickness of bag less than 0.5 cm) to insure rapid heat transfer, placed in a programmable freezer and frozen at 1°C/min from 0 to −80°C. After freezing the bags are transferred to cannisters for inventory purposes and stored in the vapor or liquid phase (less than 160°C) of liquified nitrogen. Preservation of viability appears to improve with storage in these conditions as opposed to less cold conditions [28]. In the cryopreserved state kept in optimal storage conditions, stem cell viability remains adequate for up to 3 years. Longer periods of storage have not been clinically evaluated. Bone marrow has also been adequately preserved in the liquid state at 4°C for periods of 48 hours or less [29].

3.4. Marrow reinfusion

DMSO, in the amount necessary for cryoprotection given intravenously is nontoxic [30]. In addition, rapid membrane transport of the drug enables rapid thawing and dilution before intravenous administration. Although rapid thaw is preferred by most investigators, dilution can be rapid or gradual [31]. In our institution, the bone marrow is thawed at the patient's bedside and rapidly administered intravenously. Complications to marrow infused are transient nausea, vomiting and flushing all presumed due to the DMSO.

3.5. Assessment of marrow viability

Unfortunately, no satisfactory assay for the pluripotential marrow stem cell in man exists and therefore no direct measurement of the reconstitutive capacity is available. More committed progenitor cells such as the CFC gemm or CFC gm have been cultured *in vitro* and evaluated as measures of marrow viability and reconstitutive capacity [32]. The lack of standardization of these assays and the biologic variability in growth may limit the usefulness of this assay.

The ultimate demonstration of adequate stem cell viability after cryopreservation is the ability of the transplanted marrow to reconstitute hematopoiesis in man after marrow ablative therapy. Total body irradiation with chemotherapy fulfills the requirement of marrow ablative therapy [33]. Using cyclophosphamide or piperizenedione and total body irradiation, two groups have adequately reconstituted hematopoiesis with cryopreserved remission marrows of patients with leukemia and lymphoma [34, 35]. In one study, in patients with lymphoma (and presumably normal marrow stem cells), hematologic recovery was similar to that of fresh syngeneic marrow transplants [36]. Leukemia patients had longer intervals for recovery. Table 2 summarizes this data [34, 35].

Although other studies using high-dose combination chemotherapy exhibited hematologic recovery in a similar range [4], without the knowledge that the patient's marrow was ablated, one cannot unequivocally accept that

Table 2. Hematologic recovery after ABMTX.

		Days after transplant to	
	No. patients	Neutrophils $> 500/\mu l$	Platelets $> 20,000/\mu l$
Acute leukemia	11	21 (15–35)[b]	22 (20–80)
	11	35 (20–44)[a]	34 (13–127)
Lymphoma	12	20 (11–37)[a]	23 (12–40)
Syngeneic (fresh)	16	16 (12–33)[a]	19 (8–36)

[a] Median, parenthesis indicate range [34].
[b] Mean, parenthesis indicate range [35].

complete reconstitution of hematopoiesis was accomplished solely by the transplanted marrow.

The quantity of nucleated cells required for marrow reconstitution has not been directly determined in man. 3×10^8 nucleated cells/kg are required in allogeneic transplants based on the experience with aplastic anemia [6]. However, this disease state is not ideal to evaluate hematopoiesis. Extrapolated from canine experiments using total body irradiation, and with optimal storage conditions, approximately $0.2-0.5 \times 10^8$/kg cells are required for human autologous marrow reconstitution [37].

4. CLINICAL APPLICATION OF ABMTX

There are two basic study designs for the application of ABMTX in cancer therapy. One approach is the use of existing effective standard combination chemotherapy regimens with empiric escalations of myelosuppressive drugs to 'high-dose' levels. Presumably, this intensive regimen would require ABMTX to either shorten the duration of myelosuppression or reconstitute completely ablated marrow in the patient. The advantage of this approach is the assumption that since the standard dose combination is effective, dose escalations should further augment activity. However, the empiric escalation technique has limitations. Although some agents such as ionizing radiation [38], cyclophosphamide [39], BCNU [40] and mitomycin C [41] have established acute dose limitations due to extramedullary toxicities, many agents have not been adequately studied. Thus, empiric escalations might use a drug at less than maximal dose and not achieve full cytotoxic benefit. In addition, toxic synergistic reactions from the combination might not be predicted or implicated making subsequent dose adjustments arbitrary. The empiric approach would be a 'hit or miss' attempt to augment therapeutic efficacy without beforehand knowledge of the toxicity.

The second approach would use the traditional scheme of drug development [42]. Single myelosuppressive agents would each be studied to determine new dose limits since ABMTX abrogates myelotoxic dose restraints (Phase I study). Then these agents at the maximal tolerated dose would be evaluated against a broad array of tumors (Phase II study) to define antitumor activity. Presumably these high-dose agents would show augmented activity against tumors which are responsive to the agent at standard dose and also possibly demonstrate novel tumor activity at the high-dose level. Eventually, high-dose agents with nonoverlapping extramedullary toxicities and similar antitumor activity would be combined in high doses to be compared in activity against standard regimens (Phase III study). This scheme would use each agent at a defined high dose with known toxicities. This approach would require considerable developmental time but might reveal novel therapeutic efficacy. In addition, toxicity would be more predictable than in empiric escalations minimizing unanticipated prohibitive extramedullary toxicities.

The two previous schemas have used high-dose therapy with ABMTX as sole therapy. Other considerations would be sequential use of high-dose therapy and standard therapy. This approach has appeal since the prolonged interval necessary for hematopoietic recovery after transplantation and consequently long intervals between courses might allow for substantial tumor regrowth. Although some tumors such as Burkitt's lymphoma and acute leukemia can be erradicated by one course of intense therapy, other less responsive neoplasms might require multiple courses. Thus high-dose therapy could be used as intense induction (as in acute leukemia) followed by standard consolidation therapy, or intermittently with standard therapy or as late intensification after the maximal benefit of standard therapy (i.e. the Norton-Simon hypothesis [43]).

A last approach for ABMTX would be to restore hematopoiesis after aggressive standard chemotherapy. For example, instead of initiating each course of standard therapy after hematopoietic recovery, one could administer courses at a fixed interval. This interval should be short enough not to allow for any tumor regrowth. If full hemotopoietic recovery was not achieved between each course of therapy, ABMTX after the last course would restore full hematopoiesis.

However, considering the potential limitations and alternative uses of ABMTX, the ultimate approach would be development of cytoreductive therapy of such magnitude that only a single course of therapy be required.

5. HIGH-DOSE STUDIES IN LUNG CANCER

Small cell carcinoma of the lung is a prototype tumor for which high-dose therapy has been applied because of the high response rate and near eradication with standard therapy [44]. For example, Martin and co-workers treated patients with CCNU, cyclophosphamide and methotrexate. Randomization was between a 'standard dose' scheme and a 'high-dose' scheme [45]. Doses in the high-dose scheme were two times greater than the standard therapy. A response rate of 96% (30% complete, 66% partial) was achieved with the high doses compared to 30% (30% partial, 0% complete) using standard doses. Although the doses in the high-dose regimen were only moderate compared to transplantation type doses, the higher complete response rate suggests dose-response benefits. Since small cell carcinoma of the lung responds to myelosuppressive agents such as alkylating agents, ionizing radiation, doxorubicin and the nitrosoureas, high-dose regimens using these active agents have been tried at large institutions experienced in allografting and autografting. The University of Washington at Seattle treated patients with cyclophosphamide, total body irradiation (TBI) and BCNU but found it too toxic [46]. UCLA tried a multi-agent regimen including vinblastine, cyclophosphamide, doxorubicin, methotrexate and TBI that produced severe pulmonary and cardiac toxicity [5]. The Johns Hopkins group reported only a brief partial response in one patient treated with two five-day courses of cyclophosphamide, doxorubicin, VP16-213 followed by 800 rads of TBI [47]. The largest series was performed by M.D. Anderson Hospital using a combination of cyclophosphamide 1500 mg/m^2/day for 3 days, VP16-213, 200 mg/m^2/day for 3 days, doxorubicin 80 mg/m^2/day and vincristine 1.5 mg/m^2/day for two days [48]. The combination was given twice, followed by reinfusion of cryopreserved marrow. Acute cardiac arrythmias forced the deletion of doxorubicin from some courses. After completion of this intense induction, prophylactic cranial irradiation followed by thoracic irradiation to the primary tumor was accomplished. Then, maintenance chemotherapy using the same drugs in standard doses were applied. Limited and extensive stage patients were treated with an overall response rate of 100 % (54 % complete). The complete response for limited patients was 62 % (5/8) *vs* 40 % for extensive patients (2/5). The median survival was 54 weeks with only one limited patient in sustained remission at 83 weeks. Toxicity was marrow suppression, nausea, vomiting, mucositis and fever. Unfortunately, although increasing toxicity, this study fails to depart from the results using standard therapy. The helter-skelter nature of these combinations with profound toxicities and disappointing results suggests the possible limitations of high-dose therapy.

Single agent trials in previously treated patients with small cell carcinoma have been tried using high-dose BCNU. Brief partial responses without patient benefit were seen in most patients [40]. One of the most provocative single agent studies was performed at the University College Hospital of London [49]. Sixteen patients with untreated small cell carcinoma (13 limited, 3 extensive) were treated with one course of cyclophosphamide 160–200 mg/kg followed by ABMTX. Tumor assessment was made after hematologic recovery. Then conventional irradiation to the primary tumor was administered. Eleven patients had complete responses, 2 had partial responses and 3 no responses. Seven of the complete responders are disease-free 30 to 70 weeks later. Although a preliminary report without long-term follow-up, the brevity of therapy resulting in a complete response of 69 % supports a dose-response relationship since the response to standard dose cyclophosphamide is only 28 % [50].

At Vanderbilt University, escalations of VP16-213 with ABMTX have been performed in a variety of neoplasms. From our data in ambulatory patients, VP16-213 at 1200 mg/m^2 does not produce a degree of marrow suppression to warrant ABMTX. Thirteen patients with extensive SCCL were treated with two courses of VP16-213 at 1200 mg/m^2, followed by standard cyclophosphamide, doxorubicin and vincristine with thoracic irradiation. After six courses of standard chemotherapy a final course of VP16-213 at 1200 mg/m^2 was given. Of 10 ambulatory patients, 8 had good responses to VP16-213. Follow-up is too brief to define survival but the preliminary response rate after higher-dose VP16 is twice that anticipated with standard dose VP16-213 [50].

Non-small cell carcinoma of the lung has been infrequently studied with high-dose therapy since no effective standard therapy is available to suggest agents for dose escalation studies.

6. SUMMARY AND CONCLUSIONS

BMTX has added a new dimension to cancer therapy by allowing intensification of cytotoxic therapy. Although initially limited to histocompatible siblings, the development of cryopreservation techniques has allowed autologous transplants. By using a patient as both marrow donor and recipient, ABMTX avoids the necessity of having a histocompatible donor and pretransplant immunosuppression. In addition, graft-*vs*-host disease should not occur. Although extensive laboratory evidence is available to support a dose-response relationship with therapy and cytotoxic effect, only recently have clinical studies supported that *in vitro* observation. For example, high-dose therapy with cyclophosphamide and TBI with ABMTX have cured refractory patients with lymphoma after one course of therapy and prolonged survivors are described in small cell carcinoma of the lung and testicular carcinoma using intense regimens [34, 35]. In carcinoma of the lung only a few preliminary studies are available. Empiric high-dose combinations have generally been toxic with no improvement over standard therapy. Approaches using high-dose single agents with ABMTX and sequential standard and high-dose therapy are being performed. With the proliferation of centers capable of cryopreserving and transplanting marrows, more critical studies should soon be available to better define the value of high-dose therapy in lung cancer.

ACKNOWLEDGMENT

This work was supported by a grant from the Kleberg Foundation. The author is the recipient of an American Cancer Society Junior Clinical Faculty Fellowship.

REFERENCES

1. Johnson FL, Thomas ED, Clark BS, et al.: A comparison of marrow transplantation with chemotherapy for children with ALL in second or subsequent remissions. NEJM 305: 846–851, 1981.
2. Thomas ED, Buckner CD, Clift RA, et al.: Marrow transplantation for acute nonlymphocytic leukemia in first remission. NEJM 301: 597–599, 1979.
3. Goldman JM, Catavsky D, Galton DAG: Reversal of blast cell crisis in CGL by transfusion of stored autologous buffy coat cells. Lancet 1:437–433, 1978.
4. Applebaum FR, Herzig GP, Ziegler JL, et al.: Successful engraftment of cryopreserved autologous bone marrow in patients with malignant lymphoma. Blood 52:85–95, 1978.
5. Douer D, Champlin RR, Mo W, et al.: High-dose combined modality therapy and ABMTX in resistant cancer. Am J Med 71:973–976, 1981.
6. Storb R, Thomas ED, Buckner CD: Marrow transplantation in thirty 'untransfused' patients with severe aplastic anemia. Annals of Int Med 92:30–36, 1980.
7. Coccia PF, Kriviti W, Carvenka J, et al.: Successful bone marrow transplantation for infantile malignant osteopetrosis. NEJM 302:701–703, 1980.
8. Slavini RE, Santos GW: The graft versus host reaction in man after bone marrow transplantation: Pathology, pathogenesis, clinical features and implications. Clin Imm and Immunopath 1:472–498, 1973.
9. Gaydos L, Freireich E, Mantel N: The quantitative relationship between platelet count and hemorrhage in patients with acute leukemia. NEJM 266:905–909, 1962.
10. Boggs DR: Transfusion of neutrophils as prevention or treatment of infection in patients with neutropenia. NEJM 290:1055–1062, 1974.
11. Blum RH, Frei III E: Combination chemotherapy. In: Methods in Cancer Research, Vol XVII Cancer Drug Development, Part B. DeVita V. Bush H (eds). New York: Academic Press, 1979, pp 215–257.
12. Frei III E, Canellos GP: Dose: A critical factor in cancer chemotherapy. Am J of Med 69:535–594, 1980.
13. Bruce WR, Meeker BE, Valeriote FA: Comparison of the sensitivity of normal hematopoietic and transplanted lymphoma colony-forming cells to chemotherapeutic agents administered in vivo. J Nat Cancer Inst 37:233–245, 1966.
14. Kaplan HS: Evidence for a tumoricidal dose used in the radiotherapy of Hodgkin's disease. Cancer Res 26:1221–1228, 1966.
15. Peacock JH, Stephen TC: Influence of anaesthetics on tumor-cell kill and repopulation in BI6 melanoma treated with melphalan. Br J Cancer 33:725–731, 1973.
16. Moseley MS, Eilber FR, Morton D: Melanoma in: Cancer treatment. Haskell CM (ed). Philadelphia: WB Saunders, 1980, pp 678–694.
17. McElwain TJ, Medley DW, Gordon MY, et al.: High dose melphalan and non-cryopreserved autologous bone marrow treatment of malignant melanoma and neuroblastoma. Exp Heam 7: supl: 5, 362–371, 1979.
18. Thatcher CJ, Walker IG: Sensitivity of confluent and cycling embryonic hamster cells in

sulfur mustard, 1.3-bis(chloroethyl)-1-nitrosourea and actinomycin D. J Natl Cancer Inst 42:363–363, 1969.

19. Fay JW, Levine MN, Philips GL, et al.: Treatment of metastatic melanoma with intensive BCNU and autologous bone marrow transplantation. Proc AACR/ASCO 22:532, 1931.

20. Strifei RJ, Jardke I: Analysis of the anticancer drug VP16-213 and VM 26 and their metabolites by HPLC. J of Chrom 132:211–220, 1980.

21. Wolff SN: (manuscript in preparation).

22. Wolff SN, Fer ME, McKay C, et al.: High-dose VP16 and autologous bone marrow transplantation for advanced malignancies – a phase I study. Proc AACR 23:134, 1982.

23. Chabner BA: Pharmacologic considerations in autologous bone marrow transplant regimens. In: Biology of Bone Marrow Transplantation. Gale RP and Fox CF (eds). New York: Academic Press, 1980, pp 137–144.

24. Chabner BA, Meyers CE, Oliverio VT: Clinical pharmacology of anticancer drugs. Sem Oncol 4:165–192, 1977.

25. Abrams RA, Johnston-Early A, Kramer C, et al.: Amplification of circulating granulocyte-monocyte stem cell numbers following chemotherapy in patients with extensive small cell carcinoma of the lung. Cancer Res 41:35–41, 1981.

26. Gorin NC, Muller JY, Salmon CH, et al.: Immunocompetence following ABMTX. Exp Hema 7 (supps) 327–346, 1979.

27. Ashwood-Smith MJ, Farrant J (eds).: Low Temperature Preservation in Medicine and Biology. Baltimore: University Park Press, 1980.

28. Malinini TL, Pegg DE, Perry VP, et al.: Long-term storage of bone marrow cells at liquid nitrogen and dry ice temperatures. Cryobiol 7:65–69, 1970.

29. Mangalik A, Robinson WA, Drebin C: Liquid storage of bone marrow. Exp Hema 7 (sup 5) 76–94, 1979.

30. Kligman AM: Topical pharmacology and toxicology of dimethyl sulfoxide. JAMA 193:140–156, 1965.

31. McGann LE, Turner AR, Allalunis MJ, et al.: Cryopreservation of human peripheral blood stem cells: Optimal cooling and warming condition. Cryobiol 18:469–472, 1981.

32. Fauser AA, Messner MA: Proliferative state of human pluripotent hemopoietic progenitors (CFU-GEMM) in normal individuals and under regenerative conditions after bone marrow transplantation. Blood 54:1197–1200, 1979.

33. Hager EB, Mannick JA, Thomas ED, et al.: Dogs that survive lethal exposures to radiation. Radiation Res 14:192–205, 1961.

34. Herzig GP: Autologous marrow transplantation in cancer therapy. In: Progress in Hematology, Volume XII. Brown E (ed). New York: Grune and Stratton, 1981, pp 1–25.

35. Dicke KA, Spitzer G, Peters L, et al.: Autologous bone marrow transplantation in relapsed adult acute leukemia. Lancet 1:514–517, 1979.

36. Fefer A, Einstein AB, Thomas ED, et al.: Bone marrow transplantation for hematologic neoplasia in 16 patients with identical twins. NEJM 290:1339–1393, 1974.

37. Applebaum FR, Herzig GP, Graw RG: Study of cell dose and storage time on engraftment of cryopreserved autologous bone marrow in a canine model. Transpl 26: 245–248, 1978.

38. Hellman S: Principles of radiation therapy. In: Cancer, Principles and Practice of Oncology. DeVita V, Hellman S, Rosenberg S (eds). Philadelphia: Lippincott, 1981, pp 103–131.

39. Gottdieneri JS, Applebaum FR, Ferrarsi V, et al.: Cardiotoxicity associated with high-dose cyclophosphamide therapy. Arch Int Med 141:753–563, 1981.

40. Phillips GL, Foy JW, Herzig GP, et al.: Phase I-II study: Intensive BCNU and ABMTX for refractory cancer. Cancer (in press).

41. Lazarus HM, Gottfried MR, Herzig RH, et al.: Veno-occlusive disease of the liver after high-dose mitomycin C therapy and ABMTX. Cancer (in press).

42. Methods in Cancer Research, Vol XVII Cancer Drug Development, Part B. DeVita Jr, Busch M (eds). New York: Academic Press, 1979.
43. Norton L, Simon S: Tumor size, sensitivity to therapy and design of treatment schedules. Can Tr Rep 61:1307–1317, 1977.
44. Greco FA, Oldham RK: Current concepts in cancer. Small cell lung cancer. NEJM 301:355–358, 1979.
45. Martin H, Cohen S, Craver PJ, Fossleck BF, *et al.*: Intensive chemotherapy of small cell bronchogenic carcinoma. Can Tr Rep 61:349–354, 1977.
46. Stewart PS: (personal communication).
47. Kaizer H, Whoram LL, Munor RJ, *et al.*: ABMTX in the treatment of selected human malignancies: The Johns Hopkins Oncology Center Program. Exp Hema 7: (supp 5) 309–320, 1979.
48. Farha P, Spitzer G, Valdivieso M, *et al.*: High dose chemotherapy of small cell lung cancer (manuscript in preparation).
49. Souhami RL, Herper PG, Lindi D, *et al.*: High dose cyclophosphamide with ABMTX as initial treatment of small cell carcinoma of the bronchus. Cancer Chemotherapy and Pharm (in press).
50. Minna JD, Higgins GA, Glatstein E: Cancer of the lung. In: Cancer, Principles and Practice of Oncology. DeVita V, Hellman S, Rosenberg S (eds). Philadelphia: Lippincott, 1981, pp 396–474.

6. Diagnosis of Poorly Differentiated Carcinoma of the Lung

JOHN M. LUKEMAN and BRUCE MACKAY

1. POORLY DIFFERENTIATED LUNG CARCINOMAS

Current classifications of lung cancer are based upon the morphologic patterns and cytologic features of the tumors, and the degree of cell differentiation can in addition be used in histologic grading. The four main categories recognized in most classifications, including the recent (1977) revision [1] of the 1967 World Health Organization nomenclature [2], are squamous carcinoma, adenocarcinoma, undifferentiated large cell carcinoma and undifferentiated small cell carcinoma. The better differentiated squamous and adenocarcinomas can be recognized by the pathologist with little difficulty when acceptable material for light microscopy is available. In contrast, poorly differentiated and undifferentiated tumors are open to the subjective impression of the examiner and may be designated by a variety of makeshift terms such as unclassified malignant neoplasm and anaplastic carcinoma reflecting frustration with neoplasms that do not demonstrate distinct cytomorphologic features. The degree of distortion that is often present in small biopsies is undoubtedly a major contributing factor to this lack of specificity in the labelling of lung tumors, but criteria for identifying the poorly differentiated and undifferentiated carcinomas are not well defined, and it is hardly surprising that problems constantly arise in the evaluation of small, distorted biopsies. Imprecise designations appear in pathology reports of lung neoplasms with a degree of frequency that significantly impairs the accuracy of clinico-pathologic studies, yet the pathologist who honestly attempts to append a more specific label to as many tumors as possible is likely to find that colleagues reviewing the cases will produce varying interpretations.

With the increasing use of multiple therapeutic modalities in the management of lung cancer patients, precision in the diagnosis of the tumors is of considerable importance, and the objective of this paper is to briefly review

Greco, FA (ed), Biology and Management of Lung Cancer. ISBN 0-89838-554-7.
© *1983, Martinus Nijhoff Publishers, Boston. Printed in The Netherlands.*

criteria for the cytologic, histologic and ultrastructural identification of the four major categories of lung carcinoma. Carcinoid tumors are also considered, since they frequently enter into the differential diagnosis, but mesotheliomas, the uncommon primary mesenchymal neoplasms, and metastatic tumors are omitted.

2. TISSUE PROCUREMENT

Technical problems, including inaccessibility of lesions and the hazards of taking large biopsies at endoscopy, are the main reasons that many attempted pathologic studies of lung tumors are not diagnostic. To these must be added a lack of awareness on the part of some surgeons and nurses of the importance of handling tissues gently and fixing them promptly. Alterations in the tissue prior to biopsy also contribute: biopsies taken with the flexible fiberoptic bronchoscope usually measure about 1 mm and the instrument only samples the surface of the tumor which is often distorted. Fine needle biopsies aspirate the least cohesive parts of a tissue, and necrotic areas are more likely to yield their cells than viable parts of a tumor. When a second aspirate is taken through a skinny needle without repositioning the tip, it consists largely or entirely of peripheral blood cells. Compressed or squashed cells in small biopsies may look more like fibers than neoplastic cells [3] and freezing and drying compound the problem. Artifactual change may cause cells of a differentiated primary lung carcinoma to shrink to the point where they closely simulate those of a small cell undifferentiated tumor, and this is a common source of error in diagnosis. An accurate assessment may not be possible in as many as 20% of lung and mediastinal biopsies.

Malignant cells in sputum, bronchial brushings or washings, or aspiration biopsies represent only a small sampling of a tumor, and they may not indicate the major component of a tumor that is composed of more than one cell type: this occurs more frequently than many suspect. Cytology specimens that are smeared and then air-dried show so much distortion that interpretation is often impossible. For fine needle aspiration biopsies, a mixture of equal parts of 50% ethyl alcohol and Ringer's solution is suitable if there is to be less than 2 hours delay prior to processing; otherwise, Mucolexx is excellent. In the case of fluids and brushings, it may be necessary to lyse the erythrocytes, and the specimen must then be concentrated properly, spread evenly and stained with care to allow proper comparison between normal, reactive and malignant cells. The cytoplasmic counterstain should not be too pale.

From these comments, it should be evident that we regard effective tissue procurement as an essential preliminary to the evaluation of preparations of all lung tumors, and of critical importance where the tumor is poorly differentiated. It is appropriate to add that the pathologist sampling a resection specimen should select tissue from several regions of the tumor, immerse thin (3 mm) slices promptly in 10% buffered formalin for light microscopy and, routinely, place at least one even thinner (1 mm) slice in buffered glutaraldehyde for electron microscopy. Formalin is a poor second choice for ultrastructural tissue specimens, but it may prove to be acceptable if glutaraldehyde is not available when the specimen is grossed.

3. POORLY DIFFERENTIATED ADENOCARCINOMA

Acinar formation, the hallmark of an adenocarcinoma, becomes decreasingly evident with loss of differentiation (Figure 1), but in its absence a poorly differentiated tumor may be identified as adenocarcinoma by the demonstration of cytoplasmic mucin, or from the features of the cells in tissue sections or cytologic peparations. It is possible to encounter an occasional mucin-forming cell within a squamous carcinoma, so this is not an

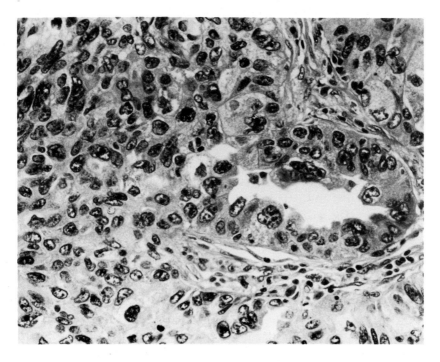

Figure 1. Tissue section of adenocarcinoma showing dedifferentiation of the cells adjacent to a gland. Note the cell pleomorphism. H & E × 360.

90

absolute criterion. Acinar formation may be confined to small zones of a poorly differentiated adenocarcinoma, and there is a better chance of encountering minute foci if multiple sections from the available blocks, and ideally sections from several areas of the tumor, are examined. An adenocarcinoma made up of sheets of uniform cells that are consistently mucin-negative may not be distinguishable from a poorly differentiated squamous carcinoma. The clinical consequences of an error at this level of dedifferentiation are not known and may be insignificant. Sharply circumscribed groups of cells are seen in both tumors though they are more common in adenocarcinomas. The occurrence of clear cells favors adenocarcinoma [4], and zones of pleomorphic cells are also more common in adenocarcinoma.

In cytologic preparations, the cells of poorly differentiated adenocarcinomas tend to be loosely cohesive. They may cluster in twos and threes or present as single cells. Aggregates of cells with a distinct community border are seldom found. Cell cohesiveness can, however, be an important diagnostic feature for adenocarcinoma in the small number of cases in which it occurs. In its absence, single cells may be diagnostic (Figure 2). The cells are usually oval and small (15–25 micrometers in diameter), though some are

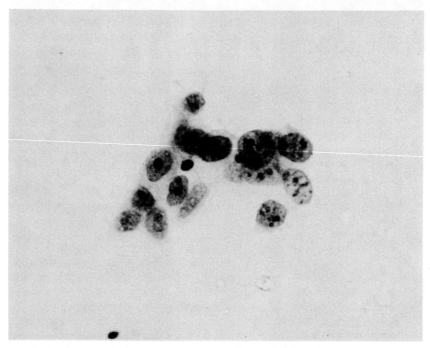

Figure 2. Cells of poorly differentiated adenocarcinoma in sputum have scanty cytoplasm, round nuclei and prominent nucleoli. × 800.

larger, and in the small cells the nuclear-cytoplasmic ratio is correspondingly high. Regardless of the degree of differentiation, adenocarcinoma cells commonly show a thin, regular nuclear membrane. The chromatin is typically clear, finely granular and weakly basophilic. Nucleoli vary and may be single and prominent or multiple and less conspicuous.

At the ultrastructural level, a poorly differentiated adenocarcinoma may display evidence of acinar formation in the presence of lumens bordered by cells with apical microvilli and joined by tight junctions. A very small lumen that would be totally unsuspected in paraffin sections will be obvious with the electron microscope. Some apparently solid carcinomas turn out to have numerous small lumens, or even mere clefts between the cells into which microvilli project. The microvilli may be uniform and straight but they do not usually contain microfilament cores like those of intestinal carcinomas. More often, the microvilli are short and curved, particularly when they project into a thin gap between adjacent cells. Apart from the tight junctions, which are not always seen in a poorly differentiated adenocarcinoma, the cells are joined by desmosomes that vary in size and number but are smaller and usually fewer than those of a squamous carcinoma. Simi-

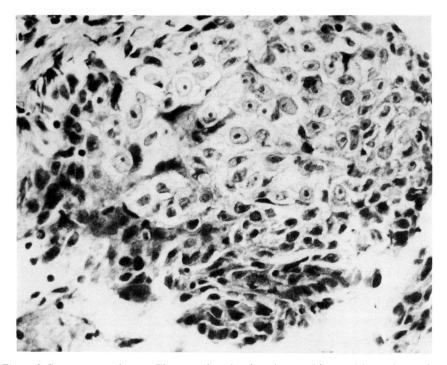

Figure 3. Squamous carcinoma. Tissue section showing pleomorphism and hyperchromasia of surface cells. Cells in the center of the lobule show nuclear irregularity and prominence of nucleoli. H & E × 450.

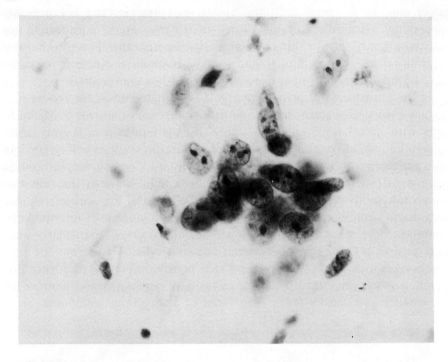

Figure 4. Sputum with cells of poorly differentiated squamous carcinoma. The cells are small, cytoplasm is fragile and nuclei show marked hyperchromasia. Nuclear detail is frequently obscured by degenerative changes. × 800.

larly, tonofilament bundles are better developed in a squamous carcinoma, though they may be present in occasional cells of an adenocarcinoma and their presence certainly should not exclude that diagnosis. Small quantities of secretory material such as mucopolysaccharides can be detected by electron microscopy within cells of tumors which, in paraffin sections, appear mucin-negative.

4. POORLY DIFFERENTIATED SQUAMOUS CARCINOMA

The cells of a poorly differentiated squamous carcinoma are usually small with scanty basophilic cytoplasm and considerable variation in nuclear size and shape (Figure 3). They typically stratify, but may form irregular cords or nests. Small groups of better differentiated cells with recognizable intercellular bridges may be found after a search of a number of areas.

In cytologic preparations, including sputum and most aspirations, the cells occur singly or in small groups. Infrequently, a few tissue fragments are encountered in an aspiration biopsy smear. As is the case in tissue sections, the cells are usually smaller than in the more differentiated tumors, and the cytoplasm is often scanty (Figure 4). Nuclei are hyperchromatic, and show more variability in size and contour than those of poorly differentiated adenocarcinomas. The nuclear membranes of the latter are usually smooth and regular and the chromatin is finely granular or even clear, in contrast to those of the squamous cells. It may, however, be extremely difficult or impossible to differentiate between a poorly differentiated squamous carcinoma and adenocarcinoma by light microscopy, since they can overlap to a considerable degree in their histologic and cytologic features. Nuclear debris and infiltration of macrophages, lymphocytes and neutrophils, and zones of frank necrosis, are characteristic of both. Occasionally the presence of tiny vacuoles in the cytoplasm of adenocarcinoma cells is helpful, and these cells sometimes have two similar appearing, overlapping nuclei, an uncommon finding in squamous carcinoma.

Varying degrees of squamous differentiation may be detected at the ultrastructural level in cells of poorly differentiated squamous carcinoma

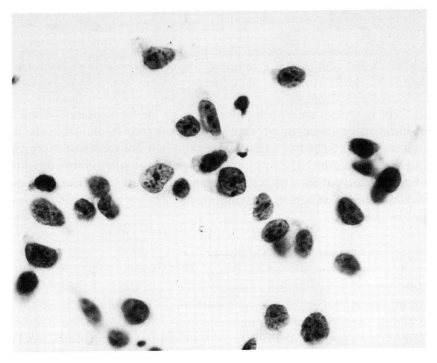

Figure 5. Aspiration biopsy of a poorly differentiated carcinoma shows epithelial cells of intermediate size with scanty cytoplasm, finely granular nuclear chromatin and rarely a prominent nucleolus. × 800.

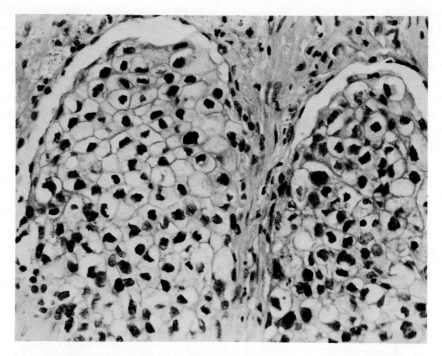

Figure 6. Poorly differentiated carcinoma. Tissue section showing tumor lobules composed of small cells with clear cytoplasm and irregular nuclei which show moderate pleomorphism and hyperchromasia. H & E × 360.

when there is no evidence of differentiation by light microscopy. They are more likely to be found in well-preserved specimens from viable areas of the tumor, and the chances of encountering them are greater if more than one area of the tumor has been sampled for electron microscopy. Frequent prominent desmosomes with associated tonofilament bundles and foci of keratin formation are squamous features.

5. POORLY DIFFERENTIATED CARCINOMA

At the present time, there is some question as to whether a category with this designation is justified. It hinges on the degree of specificity of the criteria for large cell undifferentiated carcinoma. If the latter tumor is viewed as including all dedifferentiated squamous and adenocarcinomas, then poorly differentiated carcinoma is an unnecessary term. It is not included in the revised World Health Organization classification. Nevertheless, it can be a convenient label for a carcinoma where some differentiation is suspected by light microscopy from the histologic sections or cytologic preparations, and yet the tumor cannot with any confidence be said to be either squamous carcinoma or adenocarcinoma. In these situations, electron microscopy frequently demonstrates features of one or the other. Many pathologists would include these tumors in the large cell undifferentiated category. Cytologically (Figures 5–7), the cells of poorly differentiated carcinomas are equivalent in size to those of a moderately differentiated squamous carcinoma, and the nuclei may be eccentric and irregular in profile. A moderate quantity of cytoplasm is usually visible.

6. UNDIFFERENTIATED LARGE CELL CARCINOMA

As adenocarcinomas and squamous carcinomas dedifferentiate, they progressively lose their distinctive features, and there comes a point at which these features can no longer be detected by light microscopy though there may still be evidence of the cell type at the ultrastructural level. The controversial term, poorly differentiated carcinoma, could be used for all the tumors which cannot be subclassified by light microscopy, but since they do

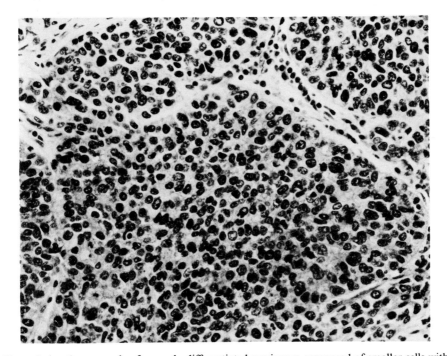

Figure 7. Another example of a poorly differentiated carcinoma composed of smaller cells with scanty cytoplasm. The cells are suggestive of oat-cell carcinoma, but by electron microscopy the tumor demonstrated features of a poorly differentiated adenocarcinoma. H & E × 360.

not display any perceptible evidence of differentiation, undifferentiated large cell carcinoma is more appropriate. If the term poorly differentiated carcinoma is retained, it becomes more difficult to define the large cell undifferentiated tumor.

If the term undifferentiated large cell carcinoma is used as a light microscopic designation for tumors showing no distinguishing features other than those of carcinoma in general, but composed of cells that differ in size and other features from small cell lung cancers, then this category will include some tumors which could be subclassified by electron microscopy. That this is the case is evident by reports of ultrastructural studies of these tumors [5, 6], in which some are shown to possess characteristics indicating that they are in fact squamous or adenocarcinomas. Since relatively few pathologists have ready access to an electron microscope for the routine study of lung tumors, it is logical to restrict the criteria to those that are reproducible and can be used by the light microscopist, aided by simple histochemical procedures such as mucin stains. More precision in subclassification is obviously possible with the use of the electron microscope, complementary to conventional optical microscopy, but there is no infor-

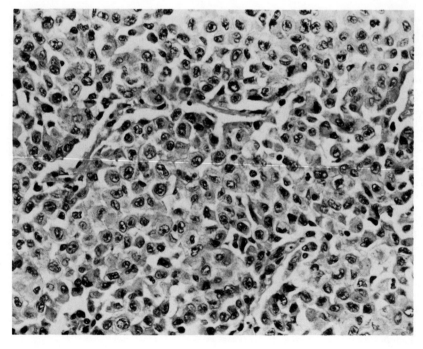

Figure 8. Undifferentiated large cell carcinoma. Tissue section showing loosely arranged cells with ample cytoplasm and prominent nucleoli. There is no evidence of an organoid pattern. H & E × 360.

mation at the present time on whether the added accuracy would significantly affect the results of clinical studies or influence patient management.

The difficulties involved in defining criteria for the identification of undifferentiated large cell carcinomas by light microscopy, and the lack of awareness of many pathologists of the significance of the category, are reflected by the occurrence of terms such as anaplastic carcinoma in the literature. There is a temptation to use this as a 'catch all' category for tumors that do not clearly fit into the other three major groups [7]. The criteria become broader if the term poorly differentiated carcinoma is retained, but in its typical form, a large cell undifferentiated carcinoma of the lung is composed of irregular aggregates of cells separated by slender connective tissue partitions. The latter are incomplete so that adjacent groups of cells communicate. Within the sheets of cells in tissue sections, the tendency is towards close apposition of the tumor cells, but areas where there is loss of cohesion can usually be found without difficulty, particularly adjacent to the zones of necrosis that are so frequent within this tumor. There are no organoid structures. If acinar formation is identified, the

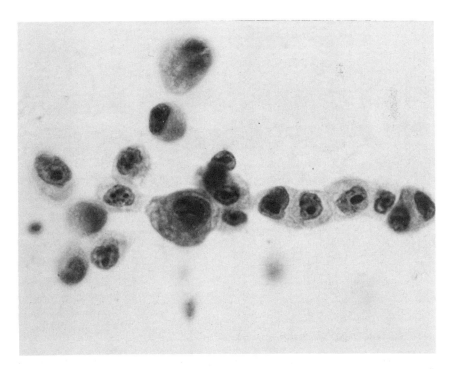

Figure 9. Cells of undifferentiated large cell carcinoma in sputum. The cytoplasm is finely vacuolated or granular. Nuclei are variable in size and nucleoli are prominent. × 800.

98

tumor is an adenocarcinoma and not a large cell undifferentiated carcinoma. The tumors cells (Figure 8) are relatively uniform, round to oval, with central round or oval nuclei that have dispersed chromatin and conspicuous nucleoli. A moderate quantity of slightly basophilic cytoplasm can be identified. In some tumors, most or all of the cells are pleomorphic, but groups of pleomorphic cells may also be encountered in more differentiated tumors, particularly adenocarcinomas [8]. The larger cells have irregular cell and nuclear profiles and some contain more than a single nucleus.

In cytologic preparations, the cells are round, oval or occasionally polyhedral, and they have ample cytoplasm. Usually there is a single round or oval nucleus which contains one or two nucleoli (Figure 9). The nuclear/cytoplasmic ratio varies from moderate to high. In good preparations, the cytoplasm may appear opaque or acidophilic, nuclear membranes are sharp, and the chromatin is finely granular. With degeneration, the nuclear shapes become more irregular and the chromatin clumps; the course granularity of the chromatin renders the nuclei hyperchromatic. In cells shed from an anaplastic tumor, giant cells with one or multiple nuclei occur sporadically, intermingled with the more regular cells depending on the composition of the tumor.

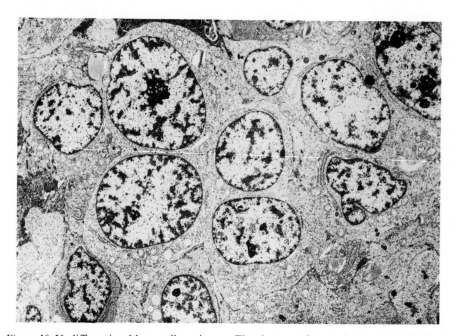

Figure 10. Undifferentiated large cell carcinoma. The electron micrograph shows several closely apposed cells with relatively high nuclear cytoplasmic ratios and sparse organelles. There is no suggestion of acinar formation, and cell junctions are inconspicuous. × 3,010.

The ultrastructural appearance of an undifferentiated large cell bronchogenic carcinoma varies to some degree depending on how stringent the light microscopic criteria for this category are. Some of the tumors to which this diagnosis is given by light microscopy will be found to possess areas of acinar formation or squamous differentiation by electron microscopy, but these are poorly differentiated tumors in which the meagre morphologic indicators of differentiation were not detected in the paraffin sections and mucin stains were negative. A truly undifferentiated tumor (Figure 10) is composed of cells with smooth, closely apposed cell membranes. The small but easily found cell junctions are desmosomes with few or no tonofilaments. Some variation in cell size and shape can be appreciated by light microscopy in semi-thin (1 micrometer) sections of the E.M. material, and with the electron microscope it is seen to be due primarily to the amount of cytoplasm. Nuclei have regular contours, fine dispersed chromatin, and usually a single large nucleolus. A moderate number of organelles including mitochondria and slender cisternae of granular endoplasmic reticulum is seen in most cells.

7. UNDIFFERENTIATED SMALL CELL CARCINOMA

The terms small cell lung cancer and oat-cell carcinoma are often used synonymously with undifferentiated small cell carcinoma. The tumor arises in the vicinity of the hilum in approximately three-fourths of cases, and the remainder occur in the mid-zone of the lung or are peripheral. A characteristic of this aggressive neoplasm is its tendency to metastasize while the primary is small and often undetected, but some tumors are large bulky masses by the time the patient seeks medical attention. Usually the cells proliferate beneath the bronchial mucosa in the early stages of growth, imparting to the bronchus a thick, shiny pipe-stem appearance. In the large tumors, extensive zones of necrosis are characteristic. Different histologic types of bronchogenic carcinoma may be associated with the production of polypeptide hormones but it is more common with the small cell tumors. A variety of hormones have been associated with this tumor [9, 10, 11] and their levels may have some role in monitoring the progress of the neoplasm.

Because of differences in biological behavior and response to therapy compared with the large cell lung tumors, identification of small cell lung cancer is of considerable clinical importance. If viable, well-preserved and processed tissue is available for study, most of these tumors can be identified by light microscopy, although some with larger cells pose a problem in distinction from large cell undifferentiated carcinomas.

The cells have a peculiar proneness to artifactual distortion that is frequently evident from the appearance of the cells in histologic and cytologic preparations. Their susceptibility to squashing is often obvious in small biopsies. This appearance is not a sine-qua-non of small cell lung cancer since it can also be seen in the more differentiated tumors and it should not, therefore, be relied upon as a diagnostic criterion.

Two of the more controversial aspects of small cell lung cancer are its histogenesis and the question of whether or not subtypes exist. The World Health Organization classification implies that subtypes can be identified by light microscopy, namely tumors composed of uniform small round cells resembling lymphocytes (oat-cell type), and tumors composed of more oval to elongated cells (intermediate variant). The validity of this subclassification has not been established, and some tumors contain areas where both cell forms can be detected. Ultrastructural studies [12] have also failed to establish criteria for subdividing the small cell lung cancers. Further studies are needed, however, in view of the occurrence of occasional long-term survivors among patients with this tumor.

Regardless of the subtype, in histologic sections the tumor cells common-

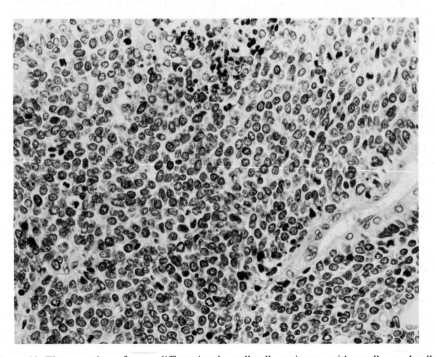

Figure 11. Tissue section of an undifferentiated small cell carcinoma with small round cells. Cytoplasm is scanty, and nuclear chromatin finely granular. Occasional nucleoli are visible. H & E × 360.

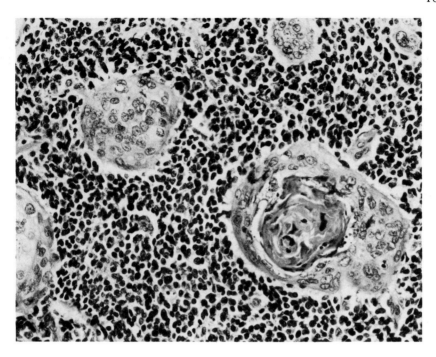

Figure 12. Tissue section of an undifferentiated small cell carcinoma showing foci of squamous differentiation. H & E × 360.

ly appear in sheets, broad cords, or aggregates without architectural patterns (Figure 11). Zones of necrosis are frequently seen and may be extensive. At the margin of the necrotic tissue, varying degrees of degenerative change within the cells are seen, and in the necrotic zones, ghost-like forms can often be identified. The hyperchromatic appearance of the tumor at low magnification is often striking and can be attributed to the relatively scanty cytoplasm and uniform nuclei of the closely packed cells.

Histologically it may be difficult to distinguish between the intermediate form of oat-cell carcinoma and a poorly differentiated adenocarcinoma. In the former tumor, cords and pseudorosettes may be present, and in some of the areas where rosette-like formations are occurring, the cells may have more cytoplasm and an impression of polarity may be conveyed by the nucleus being located towards one end of the cell. Foci of squamous differentiation (Figure 12) and areas of pseudoglandular differentiation (Figure 13) may be encountered within an otherwise pure small cell lung carcinoma.

Cytologically, the cells in sputum, aspiration biopsies, bronchial washings and brushings are similar to those in tissue sections (Figure 14), but they

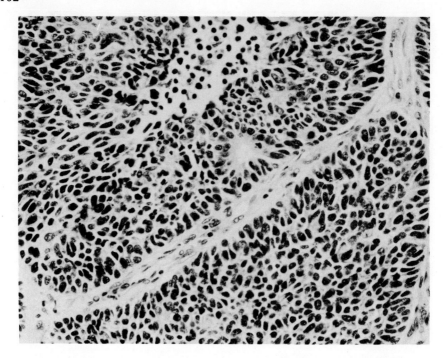

Figure 13. Tissue section of an undifferentiated small cell carcinoma showing an area of pseudoglandular differentiation. H & E × 360.

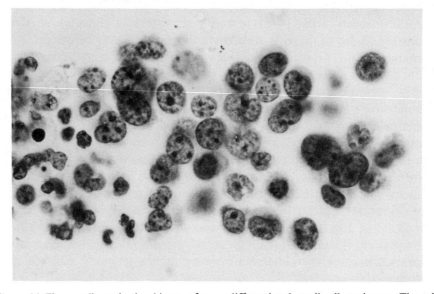

Figure 14. Fine needle aspiration biopsy of an undifferentiated small cell carcinoma. The cells rarely show intact cytoplasm, but in aspiration specimens nuclear detail is clearly demonstrated. × 800.

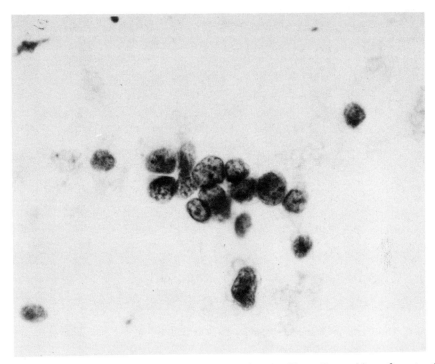

Figure 15. Sputum: undifferentiated small cell carcinoma. The cells would conform to the intermediate type, but cytologically separation from the small round cell type is difficult. The intermediate cells usually are larger, show more cytoplasm, are more elongated and their nucleoli are more prominent. × 800.

appear even more hyperchromatic, and are often found in small aggregates or in an Indian file arrangement. This tendency to aggregate is an aid in distinguishing small cell carcinoma from a malignant lymphoma since in the latter tumor the cells do not clump, mold or adhere to one another. In the intermediate form of small cell lung cancer, the cells may be 50% larger and are often less hyperchromatic than the small round, lymphocyte-like cells, and cytoplasm is readily apparent (Figures 15 and 16). Nucleoli can be observed in many of the cells. The chromatin is similar to that of the lymphocyte-like cell, and separation of the small round cell form from the intermediate type is often difficult or impossible in cytologic preparations.

Much has been made of the occurrence of dense-core granules in the cells of undifferentiated small cell carcinomas [13, 14], to the point where it is commonly stated that these tumors are dedifferentiated carcinoids. In fact, the granules are not always present, and the diagnosis must not be excluded simply because they cannot be demonstrated in a particular specimen. The

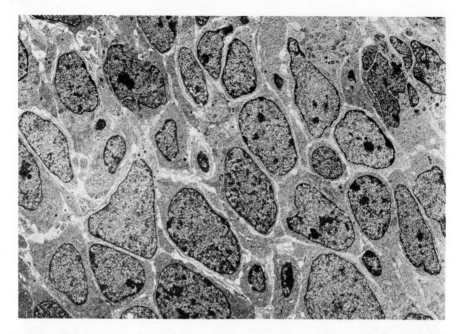

Figure 16. Undifferentiated small cell carcinoma. The cells are smaller than those of the undifferentiated large cell carcinoma shown in Figure 9, and they have very little cytoplasm. The nuclear chromatin is denser, and nucleoli are small. × 2,800.

granules are characteristically small, of the order of 150 nm in diameter, round, and clearly membrane-bound. In size they are comparable to the granules of neuroblastomas and neuroendocrine carcinomas. In contrast, most carcinoid tumors have considerable numbers of granules and they are usually more than 200 nm in diameter. There are tumors that can not be confidently placed in either category, but the majority of small cell lung cancers do not closely resemble carcinoid tumors either by light or electron microscopy.

Ultrastructurally, the cells of a small undifferentiated carcinoma of the lung vary in shape from spherical to elongated, but the majority of the tumors are composed of short oval cells (Figure 16). The nucleus is central and has a smooth profile. Chromatin is finely clumped, with the result that the nucleus is moderately electron-dense but uniform in well-preserved material, and nucleoli are usually inconspicuous. Adjacent to an area of necrosis, varying degrees of nuclear pyknosis will distort these features, and squashing has the same effect. Organelles are scanty and the cytoplasm is principally occupied by unattached ribosomes. Adjacent cells are often closely apposed, and cell junctions can be found without difficulty; they

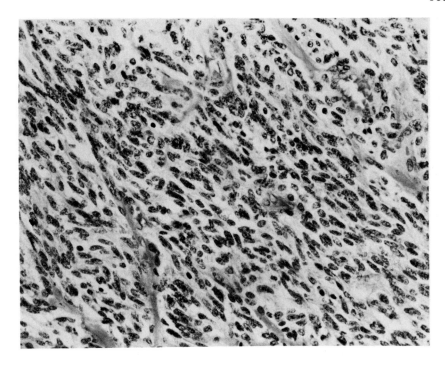

Figure 17. Spindle cell variant of a carcinoid tumor. The diagnosis was confirmed by electron microscopy. H & E × 360.

may be small desmosomes with short bundles of tonofilaments, or mere thickenings of the plasma membranes.

8. ATYPICAL CARCINOID TUMOR

Carcinoid tumor, referred to in the past as a form of bronchial adenoma, is an often indolent but potentially aggressive tumor that arises from the Kulchitsky cells of the bronchial epithelium or submucosal glands, and proliferates beneath the mucosa. Most patients are under the age of 40, in contrast to those with bronchogenic carcinoma. The tumor is composed of small, uniform, polyhedral cells with central round nuclei and moderate amounts of cytoplasm. The regular appearance of the groups of cells by light microscopy often suggests the diagnosis, but tissue biopsies are usually necessary since cells are not commonly found in induced cough specimens or sputum unless the overlying mucosa is ulcerated. Small peripheral or mid-zone nests of cells or tiny tumors (tumorlets) [15, 16] are an incidental finding in some resected lungs that show bronchiectasis or chronic pneu-

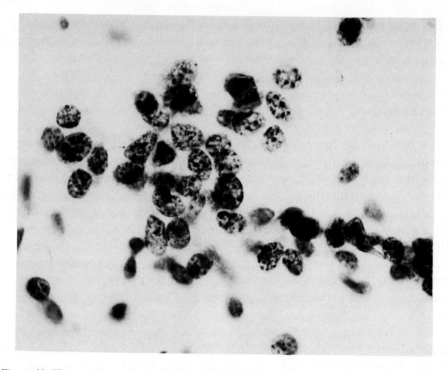

Figure 18. Fine needle aspiration biopsy of an atypical carcinoid. The cells are pleomorphic, cytoplasm is scanty and some nuclear variability can be seen. The cells resemble those of the intermediate small cell carcinoma; however, nuclear chromatin is more prominent and larger chromocenters occur. × 800.

monitis with scarring. They appear to have little propensity to spread, though occasional metastatic examples have been recorded [17].

While the typical carcinoid tumors are usually identified with little difficulty by light microscopy, problems exist with the so-called atypical forms in which the cells form diffuse sheets rather than nests, and may be oval or spindle-shaped (Figure 17). Mitotic figures are often present. In areas, the cells can simulate those of an undifferentiated small cell carcinoma. Cytologic preparations (Figure 18) are rarely effective for determining the nature of the tumor because of the low yield of cells and their similarity to cells of small cell lung cancers. The distinctive feature is the presence of cytoplasmic dense-core granules [18], and it may be possible to demonstrate them by light microscopy with the Sevier-Munger stain. They are often sparse and small, and electron microscopy is then necessary to establish the nature of the tumor. There are occasional cases where overlap in granules number and caliber render a distinction between small cell lung carcinoma and carcinoid tumor difficult or not possible, but in most instances the carcinoid cells have more and larger granules, and a greater number of cytoplasmic organelles including mitochondria, granular endoplasmic reticulum and lysosomes.

9. CONCLUSION

Problems in the diagnosis of the poorly differentiated carcinomas occur frequently when only light microscopy is employed. When necrosis is present, the cells in sputum are difficult to identify by specific cell type. A better sample with improved nuclear detail may be obtained with fine needle aspiration biopsies. Usually special histologic stains such as Alcian Blue and Mayer's Mucicarmine are not helpful in the diagnosis of the poorly differentiated tumors. Although immunologic and histochemical procedures which may help to separate the different subgroups of lung cancer are being investigated, they are still of questionable reliability and must be further evaluated. All of these tumors should be examined by electron microscopy since it is often diagnostic.

Histochemical, immunologic and enzymatic investigative procedures are daily adding to our detailed knowledge of the pathophysiologic changes that occur in premalignant and malignant tissues. Reliable staging, and improved cytologic and histologic diagnosis, coupled with modified and new therapeutic regimens are changing the survival of patients with primary lung cancers which only recently showed no or little response to therapy.

REFERENCES

1. World Health Organization: Histological Typing of Lung Tumors. Geneva: WHO 1977 (revision).
2. World Health Organization: Histological Typing of Lung Tumors. Geneva: WHO 1967.
3. Lukeman JM, Mackay B: The cytopathology and histopathology of lung cancer. Sem Resp Med 3: 140, 1982.
4. Katzenstein A-LA, Prioleau PG, Askin FB: The histologic spectrum and significance of clear-cell change in lung carcinoma. Cancer 45: 943, 1980.
5. Wang N-S, Seemayer TA, Ahmed MN, Knaack J: Giant cell carcinoma of the lung. Hum Pathol 7:3, 1976.
6. Churg A: The fine structure of large cell undifferentiated carcinoma of the lung. Hum Pathol 9:143, 1978.
7. Matthews M: Morphology of lung cancer. Sem Oncol 1:175, 1974.
8. Hathaway BM, Copeland K, Gurley J: Giant cell adenocarcinoma of the lung. Report of 21 and analysis of 139 cases. Arch Surg 98:24, 1969.
9. Gropp C, Havermann K, Scheuer A: Ectopic hormones in lung cancer patients at diagnosis and during therapy. Cancer 46:347, 1980.

108

10. Abeloff MD, Trump DL, Baylin SB: Ectopic adenocorticotrophic (ACTH) syndrome and small cell carcinoma of the lung – assessment of clinical implications in patients on combination chemotherapy. Cancer 48:1082, 1981.
11. Woo KB, Waalkes TP, Abeloff MD, Ettinger DS, McNitt KL, Gehrke CW: Multiple biologic markers in the monitoring of treatment for patients with small cell carcinoma of the lung. The use of serial levels of plasma CEA and serum carbohydrates. Cancer 48:1633, 1981.
12. Mackay B, Osborne BM, Wilson RA: Ultrastructure of lung neoplasms. In: Lung Cancer: Clinical Diagnosis and Treatment, Straus MJ (ed). New York: Grune and Stratton, 1977, p 71.
13. Fisher ER, Palekar A., Paulson JD: Comparative histopathologic, histochemical, electron microscopic and tissue culture studies of bronchial carcinoids and oat-cell carcinomas of the lung. Am J Clin Pathol 69: 165, 1978.
14. Bensch KG, Corrin B, Pariente R, Spencer H: Oat-cell carcinoma of the lung, its origin and relationship to bronchial carcinoid. Cancer 22:1163, 1968.
15. Churg A, Warnock ML: Pulmonary tumorlet. A form of peripheral carcinoid. Cancer 37:1469, 1976.
16. Ranchod M: The histogenesis and development of pulmonary tumorlets. Cancer 39:1135, 1977.
17. Hausman DH, Weimann RB: Pulmonary tumorlet with hilar lymph node metastasis. Cancer 20:1515, 1967.
18. Churg A: Large spindle cell variant of peripheral bronchial carcinoid tumor. Arch Pathol Lab Med 101:216, 1977.

7. Morphologic Changes in Small Cell Lung Cancer

MEHMET F. FER, WILLIAM W. GROSH and F. ANTHONY GRECO

1. INTRODUCTION

It is generally accepted that the morphology of malignant cells often denotes their cellular origin, predicts the natural history of the neoplasm, and therefore assists in planning therapy. Given this important role of cellular morphology in clinical oncology, observations of changing histology with time or following treatment have baffled physicians and resulted in some intriguing speculation. Changes in morphology with regard to the predominant cell type or the degree of differentiation have been observed in a variety of neoplasms [1–7]. For example, approximately one third of patients with chronic granulocytic leukemia in blast crisis will express morphologic and enzymic properties of acute lymphoblastic leukemia [1, 2]. Malignant germ cell tumors of the testicle when re-biopsied following chemotherapy will often display benign, mature teratoma histology [3, 4]. When the morphologic classification of Rappaport is used, it has been noted that many 'nodular' lymphomas eventually evolve into aggressive neoplasms with diffuse histology [5, 6]. Changes in the degree of differentiation have been well documented in medullary thyroid carcinoma and prostate cancer [7]. In both instances the time-dependent changes have implied a progressive loss of differentiating features; in the case of medullary thyroid cancer this has been associated with a decline in the production of calcitonin [7]. These observations all suggest that tumors consist of various cell populations which are subject to change with time and/or cytotoxic therapy. While adaptive processes may be involved, it is likely that pre-existing cellular heterogeneities are important [8]. The elucidation of these determinants can provide considerable insight into mechanisms by which tumors evolve, progress and become resistant to therapy.

Until effective chemotherapy became available for small cell carcinoma of the lung (SCC), all patients with metastatic lung cancer had a dismal

Greco, FA (ed), Biology and Management of Lung Cancer. ISBN 0-89838-554-7.
© *1983, Martinus Nijhoff Publishers, Boston. Printed in The Netherlands.*

prognosis and short survival. Consequently, there was little opportunity to observe changes that were time-dependent, or related to therapy. It was only in the late 1970s that morphologic alterations were observed in long-term survivors of SCC who had received intensive chemotherapy and radiotherapy, and eventually had come to autopsy [9]. Further autopsy studies and *in vitro* experiments have been subsequently performed, but information regarding the clinical features of histologic conversion is limited [10–14]. This chapter will describe the clinical experience at Vanderbilt University with changing morphology in SCC, and briefly review the literature.

2. CLINICAL EXPERIENCE WITH CHANGING MORPHOLOGY IN SCC

During the years 1976 through March of 1982, 381 patients were treated at Vanderbilt University for SCC. At least 222 of these patients are known to have relapsed and died. Approximately one fifth of all relapsing patients were re-biopsied at recurrence. Eight patients had non-SCC histologies on these repeat biopsies. One other patient was recognized after post-mortem examination. These patients were not recognized as a result of a prospective, systematic search, but reviewed retrospectively. It is likely that several more patients with changing morphology could have been detected if biopsies or autopsies were performed more frequently. The clinical features of these 9 patients are summarized in Table 1.

The clinical presentations were no different than other patients with SCC, and no predictor of morphologic conversion could be identified in retrospect. Treatment regimens for these patients have been previously described in detail [15, 16]. All chemotherapy was generally based on a combination of cyclophosphamide, doxorubicin and vincristine (CAV). Six patients with limited stage disease had received radiotherapy to the primary lesion and prophylactically to the brain. Consolidation therapy consisted of VP-16 and hexamethylmelamine, followed by methotrexate maintenance. The 3 patients with extensive stage disease received similar chemotherapy regimens: one had CAV alone, another CAV with high-dose methotrexate and a third patient had alternating cycles of CAV with VP-16, hexamethylmelamine and procarbazine. Overall 4 patients had achieved complete remission (CR) (2 limited stage, 2 extensive stage) and 5 had a partial response (4 limited stage, 1 extensive stage). One complete response was confirmed by bronchoscopy and bronchial biopsies, the others were assessed clinically and radiographically. The median duration of response was 9 months in the group, ranging from 4–45 months. Histology at relapse was purely non-SCC in 6 patients (squamous carcinoma in 5, large cell undifferentiated carcinoma in 1) but the remaining 3 patients had both SCC and non-SCC compo-

Table 1. Changing morphology in SCC: summary of patient characteristics.

Patient	Age/sex	Stage and distribution of disease at presentation	Therapy	Response and duration	Histology at relapse	Site(s) of relapse	Therapy[a] after relapse	Survival after relapse
1 JO	57/M	LS	CAV[b]	CR, 45 mo	Squamous carcinoma	Local (lung) and brain	None	5 mo
2 JM	52/F	ES	CAV	CR, 10 mo	Squamous carcinoma	Liver, brain	Methyl CCNU, procarbazine, cranial radiotherapy	5 mo
3 JR	70/M	LS	CAV	CR, 8 mo	Squamous carcinoma mixed with SCC	Lung nodules, later liver and lymph nodes	Methyl CCNU, procarbazine, CAV, VP-16, HMM	12 mo
4 WE	56/M	ES (lung, liver)	CAV with HDMTX-LV[c]	PR, 6 mo	Large cell undifferentiated carcinoma	Supraclavicular nodes, pericardium, later liver and lung	Radiotherapy to pericardium and supraclavicular areas	1 mo
5 RP	56/M	LS	CAV	PR, 8 mo	Squamous carcinoma	Bone, brain, chest wall, lung	Vindesine, later methotrexate and bleomycin	2 mo
6 JE	51/M	ES (lung, brain, bone)	CAV/VPH[d]	CR, 28 mo	Squamous carcinoma	Lung	Radiotherapy to the chest, later CCNU	6 mo
7 DL	58/F	LS	CAV	PR, 9 mo	Squamous carcinoma	Lung (later SCC in bone and bone marrow	Radiotherapy to femoral neck	7 mo

Table 1. (continued).

Patient	Age/sex	Stage and distribution of disease at presentation	Therapy	Response and duration	Histology at relapse	Site(s) of relapse	Therapy[a] after relapse	Survival after relapse
8 WS	49/M	LS	CAV	PR, 4 mo	Mixed SCC with large cell undifferentiated carcinoma, with foci of squamous (keratin+) and glandular (mucin+) differentiation	Cervical nodes, later bone and bone marrow	CAV, later VP-16, HMM, later methotrexate, procarbazine and methyl CCNU	4 mo
9 DP	66/M	LS	CMC,[e] later others	PR, 27 mo	Large cell undifferentiated carcinoma with squamous (keratin+) and glandular (mucin+) foci	Lung cervical node and bone	Vindesine, VP-16, Cis-platinum	1 mo+

Abbreviations:

LS : Limited stage (disease confined to one hemithorax and ipsilateral lymph nodes)

ES : disease spread beyond limited stage

CR : Complete response

PR : Partial response

[a] No objective response observed after relapse.

[b] Cyclophosphamide, doxorubicin, vincristin ×6 cycles, with radiotherapy to the primary lesion and prophylactically to the brain. Consolidation therapy with VP-16, hexamethylmelamine (HMM) ×3 cycles and maintenance with methotrexate ×9 cycles (described in [15] and [16].

[c] HDMTX-LV: High dose methotrexate (6 gm/m²) with leucovorin rescue.

[d] CAV alternating with VP-16, procarbazine, HMM.

[e] Cyclophosphamide, methotrexate, CCNU, followed by vinblastine, doxorubicin, and later VP-16, Cis-platinum.

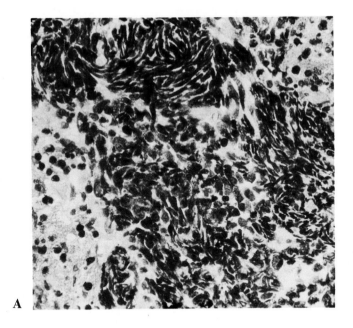

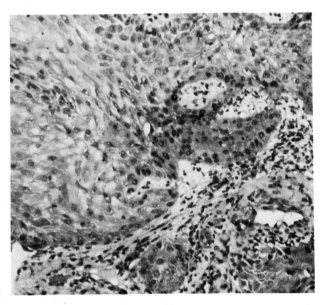

Figure 1. (A) Biopsy of mediastinal node showing small cell carcinoma; (B) Bronchial biopsy from same patient (Patient 1) at the time of relapse, demonstrating keratinizing squamous carcinoma. Small cell elements were not detected at autopsy. × 280.

nents (squamous carcinoma in 1, large cell undifferentiated carcinoma with glandular and squamous foci in 2). In one of these patients the squamous carcinoma was considered to be an incidental finding at thoracotomy which was performed for resection of a fungus ball (Patient 7, described below).

The prognosis following relapse was invariably dismal. One patient refused further therapy after recurrence, two others received radiotherapy alone and the other six received chemotherapy. These chemotherapeutic efforts are summarized in Table 1. Radiotherapy appeared to provide symptomatic relief. None of the patients responded to chemotherapy. The median survival following relapse was 4 months, ranging from 1–12 months. These patterns are no different from those observed in patients who recur with SCC histology.

Some of the patients in this series are presented below. These patients illustrate the different clinical syndromes associated with morphologic conversion in SCC.

Patient 1: J.O., a 57-year old man, presented in June 1976 with persistent epigastric discomfort. Chest X-ray revealed a right hilar mass. Sputum cytologies and bronchoscopy was negative. Mediastinoscopy in July 1976 yielded tissue diagnostic of small cell carcinoma (Figure 1A). Staging work-up was negative and he had limited stage disease. He was treated with cytoxan, adriamycin and vincristine with radiotherapy to the primary lesion and prophylactically to the brain. He achieved complete remission which continued until April of 1980 when respiratory symptoms recurred. Recurrent tumor was present in the right lower lobe and bronchial biopsies revealed squamous cell carcinoma with keratinizing cells (Figure 1B). A metastatic lesion in the calvarium was treated with radiotherapy. He declined chemotherapy. Over the ensuing months his condition deteriorated with generalized weakness, confusion, and post-obstructive pneumonia treated with multiple antibiotics. In September 1980 he died with generalized bronchopneumonia. Autopsy confirmed the presence of multiple microabscesses in both lungs, cerebral candidiasis, and squamous cell carcinoma involving the right lower lobe with no residual small cell components.

Patient 3: J.R., a 70-year old male presented with wheezing and left chest discomfort of a few months duration. Chest X-ray revealed a left hilar mass which on bronchoscopy proved to be small cell carcinoma. He had limited stage disease, treated with CAV, radiotherapy to the primary lesion and prophylactically to the brain. He achieved complete remission which continued until January of 1978 when bilateral lung nodules appeared on chest X-ray. These nodules were not accessible to noninvasive biopsy procedures and a tissue diagnosis was not pursued. Methyl CCNU and procarbazine failed to produce a response. His nodules continued to grow very slowly over several months in spite of attempts at re-induction with CAV, and later with VP-16 and hexamethylamelamine. In December of 1978, liver scan showed multiple defects compatible with metastasis. His condition declined with confusion, emaciation and chronic dyspenia. He died in February of 1979. Autopsy revealed squamous cell carcinoma in the left lower and upper lobes with metastasis to the hilar nodes. There was some keratin production. There was also a small cell component which predominantly involved the liver and retroperitoneal nodes. Microabscesses were present in the lungs. Cultures grew staph aureus and aspergillus.

Patient 6: J.E., a 51-year old male presented with confusion, headaches, and blindness which had developed over a few days. CT of the brain had revealed multiple metastatic lesions primarily in both occipital lobes. Chest X-ray revealed a right lower lobe mass which on bronchoscopy proved to be a small cell carcinoma. He received radiotherapy to the brain and was begun on chemotherapy with CAV alternating with VP-16, hexamethylmelamine and procarbazine. He achieved complete remission lasting 28 months after which a recurrent chest mass and pleural effusion developed. Bronchial biopsy confirmed squamous cell carcinoma. Radiotherapy was given to the chest and a chest tube was inserted for sclerosis of the effusion. He was stable for six months after which the chest mass began to enlarge. He was started on a trial of CCNU but died two weeks later.

Patient 7: D.L., a 58-year old female had seen her personal physician for respiratory symptoms. A right upper lobe infiltrate was noted and proven to be small cell carcinoma. She received chemotherapy with CAV and radiotherapy of the primary lesion and to the brain. Shortly after the fifth cycle of chemotherapy she developed a chronic hacking cough and low grade fever. A persistent right upper lobe infiltrate was present. Cultures and bronchoscopy failed to reveal a diagnosis. Over the following few months she remained weak and coughed chronically. A trial of antibiotics did not result in improvement. By April 1981, eight months after her initial diagnosis cavitation developed in the right upper lobe infiltrate. Thoracotomy and right upper lobe resection was performed revealing aspergillosis and a single 5-mm focus of squamous cell carcinoma in the lung parenchyma. There were no small cell elements within this tumor. She did well following surgery until November 1981 at which time she developed metastatic small cell carcinoma involving the bone and bone marrow but underwent radiation to symptomatic areas. She refused further chemotherapy. She died in January 1982.

Patient 8: W.S., a 49-year old man presented to his physician in December of 1979 with shaking chills and pleuritic chest pain. An infiltrate was present on his chest X-ray, and bronchoscopy confirmed small cell carcinoma of the intermediate subtype. He had limited stage disease and was started on therapy with CAV and radiotherapy to the primary lesion and brain. A partial response was achieved but lasted only four months after which he developed a cervical node. Lymph node biopsy showed a mixed tumor with intermediate cell elements along with large cell anaplastic carcinoma and areas of squamous and glandular differentiation. There were foci which stained for mucin and other areas contained keratin. Continued attempts at tumor control with CAV and later with VP-16 and hexamethylmelamine were without benefit. The cervical node enlarged over the ensuing two months and he developed metastasis to the bone and bone marrow. Bone marrow biopsy confirmed a mixed histology with intermediate cell and large cell undifferentiated components. A trial of methotrexate, CCNU and procarbazine was not helpful. He died in October 1980, ten months following his initial diagnosis.

3. REVIEW OF THE LITERATURE

The first observation of changing histology following cytotoxic therapy for SCC was reported in 1978 by Brereton et al. [9]. This series consisted of 21 patients who were treated at the National Cancer Institute (NCI) for SCC with intensive chemotherapy and radiotherapy, and eventually came to autopsy. Five of these patients were found to be free of tumor. Of the 16 who died with tumor, 11 had SCC, while 5 had foci of squamous carcinoma. Only 1 patient had pure squamous elements, and the other 4 had a mixture of squamous and small cell histologies.

Another large autopsy review was reported by Abeloff et al. in 1979 [10]. These authors reviewed 40 patients who came to autopsy at Johns Hopkins University Hospital following therapy for SCC. Five of these 40 patients had relapsed with non-SCC histology alone (3 squamous carcinomas, 1 adenocarcinoma and 1 large cell anaplastic carcinoma) while in another 6 patients the tumors contained non-SCC components along with SCC (4 adenocarcinomas, 1 large cell anaplastic carcinoma and 1 with squamous and glandular elements, as well as SCC). Patient histories were presented in detail. All 5 patients who eventually relapsed with non-SCC alone had presented with limited stage disease. Four patients had the intermediate subtype of SCC, and only one had the lymphocyte-like (oat cell) subtype. Three had hilar lesions on their initial chest X-ray, while 2 had apparent primary lesions in the peripheral lung field. All patients received combination chemotherapy, and 4 had radiotherapy to the primary tumor. One patient had relapsed with squamous carcinoma after a three-year complete remission of her SCC, two other patients had had a partial response and the remaining two had no response. The survival pattern in this series was better than one would expect from the natural history of SCC, and even the two nonresponders had lived 291 and 774 days. Biochemical analysis of tumor tissue obtained at autopsy indicated that despite some overlap, histaminase and dopa-decarboxylase activities in these tumors were clearly lower than those observed in SCC.

An expanded autopsy series from the NCI and the Working Party for Therapy of Lung Cancer (WP-L) was reported by Matthews in 1979 [11]. This series included the five patients originally reported by Brereton et al. Of the 97 patients with SCC who eventually came to autopsy, 35 (36%) had non-SCC elements at the time of death. All of these patients had received chemotherapy with or without radiotherapy. Five of these patients had relapsed only with non-SCC (3 anaplastic large cell carcinomas with giant cell components, 2 epidermoid carcinomas with carcinoid component) while the remaining 30 had mixed SCC and non-SCC histology (SCC with giant cell component in 12, with squamous cell component in 3, tubular component in 8, squamous and tubular components in 3, carcinoid component in 4). Clinical features were not described further in this review.

3.1. In vitro models of changing morphology

Several studies have been directed at the in vitro growth patterns of SCC. In these studies it is often observed that cellular morphology changes along with biochemical properties of the tumor cells during prolonged passage in tissue culture.

In the series reported by Gazdar et al., five of the six SCC cell culture lines maintained for 24–60 months manifested alterations in morphology [13]. In contrast, none of the 12 culture lines manifested any change within 24 months. The morphologic change was gradual. Initially 'transitional' cells appeared, which maintained the classical diffusely granular nuclear pattern of SCC but had prominent, eosinophilic nucleoli [13]. These transitional cells were eventually replaced by cells which were morphologically identical to large cell undifferentiated carcinoma. All SCC culture lines originally possessed 'amine precursor uptake decarboxylase' (APUD) cell properties, including high levels of dopa-decarboxylase, polypeptide hormone secretion, formaldehyde-induced fluorescence and neuro-secretory type granules on electron microscopy. These features were apparently retained during the 'transitional' stage, but lost when a predominantly large cell morphology was acquired [13]. Interestingly, one of these culture lines developed a mixed population of cells with SCC and squamous cell elements, and some cells manifested features characteristic of both types, such as the co-existence of tonofilaments and neuro-secretory type granules.

The same group of investigators also studied creatinine-kinase BB (CK-BB) isoenzyme as a marker of SCC in these cultures, and observed that elevated levels of CK-BB were maintained following morphologic conversion, although APUD characteristics such as dopa-decarboxylase production were lost [17]. This suggested that the measured biochemical parameters were controlled in a discordant fashion. Thus, it is again apparent that histologic conversion does not imply an 'all-or none' type change, and some features of the original phenotype may be preserved during certain stages of the process.

4. DISCUSSION

The observed morphologic conversion from SCC to non-SCC histology can be explained by one or more of the following possibilities.

1. SCC is often diagnosed by bronchoscopic biopsy, sputum cytology, and occasionally by mediastinoscopy or percutaneous needle aspiration biopsy. Since all of these methods provide a very small amount of tissue for morphologic examination, sampling errors may occur, particularly in tumors with mixed histology. Establishing the incidence of tumors with mixed histology prior to any therapy could help define this possibility. Matthews and Gazdar have reported that of 121 patients with SCC reviewed at the NCI – VA Medical Oncology Branch, 18 (14.8%) were mixed tumors with non-SCC components (WP-L type 22/40) [18]. In another series reviewed by Matthews of over 800 patients who underwent resection of lung tumors by the Veterans Administration Surgical Oncology Group, 35 had SCC [19]. Of these 35 patients, 2 had mixed tumors with non-SCC components. Bates *et al.* reported their experience in 29 patients with biopsy-proven SCC who underwent radiotherapy immediately followed by surgery [20]. These patients received 1750 rads over eight days and were taken to thoracotomy within one to seven days after completing radiotherapy. Of these 29 patients, 6 had poorly differentiated squamous carcinoma in the resected specimens. In another study by Larsson and Zettergren, 479 primary lung cancers were reviewed and the initial pathologic diagnosis was compared with that proven after excisional surgery [21]. These patients did not receive any cytotoxic therapy in the interim between their initial diagnostic procedure (bronchoscopy or mediastinoscopy) and thoracotomy. It was reported that of the 25 patients who carried an initial diagnosis of SCC, 2 were classified as squamous cell carcinoma after thoracotomy. However, the authors did not comment on the presence of mixed histology and it is possible that this limited discrepancy in the diagnosis may have been due to the inadequacy of the initial biopsy sample.

At Vanderbilt University the role of 'adjuvant surgery' is being evaluated in limited stage SCC (Dr Comis discusses this concept in detail elsewhere in this monograph). Since mid-1980, 7 patients have been taken to surgery

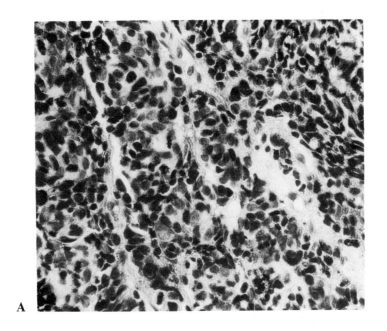

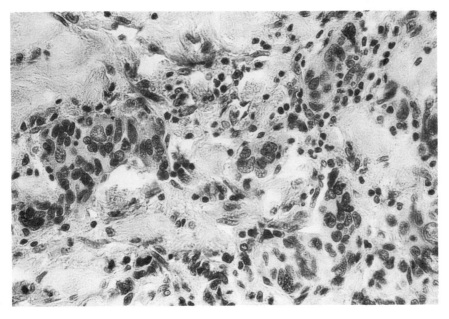

Figure 2. (A) Bronchial biopsy revealing small cell carcinoma; (B) Section of residual tumor resected after two cycles of intensive chemotherapy, showing mixed elements with large cell undifferentiated carcinoma. × 280.

120

following two cycles of intensive combination chemotherapy with cyclo-phosphamide, doxorubicin, vincristine and VP-16. Of these 7 patients, 2 were found to have large cell undifferentiated carcinoma components mixed with small cell elements within the resected specimens (Figure 2).

These findings suggest that as many as 15% of SCCs may have mixed histology at the time of initial diagnosis. It is possible that these non-small cell elements may emerge with time in patients who achieve control of their SCC.

2. Morphologic changes may evolve with time, or as a consequence of cytotoxic therapy. The *in vitro* observations of gradual and progressive transition from SCC to non-SCC that have been noted in cell cultures are particularly important, since these cells are not exposed to radiation or chemotherapy and there is no question of sampling error. These time-dependent changes challenge the notion that different histologic types of lung cancer arise from separate cells of origin, since they strongly suggest a continuous transition phenomenon between different cell types. It has been proposed that these observations are in conformity with a unified concept of histogenesis for lung cancer, which implies that different histologic types of lung cancer represent different stages in the de-differentiation spectrum [22]. Baylin and Mendelsohn suggest that tumor progression may involve some mobility within this broad histologic spectrum thus accounting for changes observed at different points in time [22]. In contrast to *in vitro* changes that occur without any interference by drugs or radiation, clinical observations of morphologic conversions have been seen only in patients undergoing cytotoxic therapy. In the absence of a 'control' group of untreated long-term survivors, the role of cytotoxic agents in inducing these changes remains speculative.

3. The two histologic types may represent independent primary tumors. This would appear unlikely in most instances, simply based on the observed low incidence of concomitant primary tumors, and the low probability that these two independent neoplasms would arise within such close proximity. This type of explanation is much more plausible in the case of prolonged survivors who develop a second lung tumor in a different location. Nevertheless, it is conceivable that if a certain portion of the bronchial tree is more susceptible to carcinogenic stimuli for whatever reason, more than one primary tumor may arise within that area. The incidence of such double primaries could be underestimated from conventional clinical reviews, since in any given case the tumor expressing the higher growth rate would most likely obscure the other. If the dominating neoplasm (which in this case would be the SCC) is eradicated by radiotherapy, the silent companion that is refractory to therapy could then become apparent.

Reports of multiple primary lung tumors have been limited. In one study,

Auerbach *et al.* performed 50–208 sections of the tracheobronchial tree in each of 255 patients who had died of primary lung cancer [23]. They found that at least 9 patients (3.5%) had other lesions compatible with multiple foci of primary lung cancer [23]. These authors indicated that if they included cases where some uncertainty existed, the incidence of multiple bronchogenic carcinomas could be as high as 14.5%. Since this report no other series have been published to expand on these observations. In a review of multiple primary lung cancers diagnosed at Memorial Hospital between 1955 to 1974, Martini and Melamed [25] found 50 such patients, among a total of 5163 bronchogenic carcinomas seen at that institution during the study period (0.97%). Since this was a retrospective surgical series, none of the first tumors were SCC. Two patients developed SCC during follow-up after resection of a non-SCC. In a literature review of histologically different multiple lung cancers, Mobley and Martinez [24] only found 33 such reported cases. These authors concluded that multiple primary lung cancers with different histology must be rare.

At Vanderbilt University, one patient (among a total of 381 patients with SCC) developed a second lung cancer with non-SCC histology, during remission of his SCC. This was a 66-year old man who presented with limited stage small cell carcinoma (oat-cell subtype), involving the right upper lobe in August 1976. He was treated with CAV, radiotherapy to the chest lesion and prophylactically to the brain, resulting in complete remission. He received consolidation therapy with VP-16, hexamethylmelamine and later methotrexate. Re-staging bronchoscopy performed in August 1977 showed squamous cell carcinoma *in situ* in the bronchial biopsies from the *left* upper lobe. There was an area of questionable submucosal invasion. He was followed without further therapy until March 1980, when he developed a chronic cough and left upper lobe infiltrate. Repeat bronchoscopy showed a fungating mass, biopsies confirming squamous carcinoma. Progression was rapid, with multiple lung metastases and overall debility. He died in May 1980, without evidence of recurrent SCC.

4. Finally, it is possible that interobserver or intraobserver variations in the interpretation of lung cancer samples may give the impression that histology may have changed, when samples obtained at different points in time are compared. It is well recognized that consistency in the histologic typing of lung cancer requires considerable experience, due to the pleomorphism of many lung tumors. Feinstein *et al.* evaluated the consistency between five independent pathologists in reading 50 lung cancer cases [26]. All pathologists gave two independent readings of each slide, so that intraobserver variations could also be determined. These authors observed that although the well-differentiated tumors could be identified consistently over 95% of the time, disagreements were more common in poorly differentiated carci-

122

nomas. Discrepancies between the first and second readings of the same tumor by the same pathologist ranged from 2 to 20% for the five pathologists. More recently, Stanley and Matthews reported much better correlation among three pathologists who independently typed 476 lung cancers [27]. At least two of the three pathologists agreed on the diagnosis in 94% of the cases. However, it was also noted that of tumors with an initial interpretation of SCC, 11% were classified as non-SCC when reviewed by the other two observers. These authors feel that when specific guidelines for classification are used, the correlation between different pathologists should be high. Nevertheless, an observation of 'changing histology' should be critically reviewed within this context, and a concensus of opinions among different observers should be sought when possible.

Certain practical conclusions can be derived from the observations described above. The potential heterogeneity of SCC should be considered when evaluating past therapeutic failures and when designing new treatment protocols. The surgical pathologist should be provided an adequate biopsy sample for a detailed examination. Whenever possible, lymph node metastases or other easily accessible tumor nodules should be biopsied and multiple sections reviewed in order to define the subset of patients with mixed histology. Although those patients should still be approached as SCC, the observed low complete remission rate in these patients may make them suitable candidates for more aggressive investigational therapy. For example, protocols incorporating surgical resection of localized tumors or radiotherapy should be considered in this population, since it is likely that non-SCC elements may be refractory to chemotherapy. Patients with SCC who relapse following chemotherapy or radiation should be biopsied whenever feasible, in order to determine possible alterations in morphology. Additionally, a variety of studies which can provide clues to distinguish SCC from non-SCC lung neoplasms can complement the descriptions of cellular morphology, and should be performed on these tumors when available. For example, certain antigens have been associated with SCC, and others with non-SCC [28, 29]. A chromosome abnormality has been recently reported for SCC (deletion 3p (14-23) [30]. Further experience which describes the *in vivo* natural history of tumors with changing morphology, along with the assessment of other biochemical, genetic and antigenic parameters may shed additional light on the biology of these neoplasms, and allow clinicians to design more rational treatment programs.

ACKNOWLEDGMENT

This work was supported in part by grants 1 R01 CA 27333 and R-25 CA 19429 from the National Cancer Institute.

REFERENCES

1. Rosenthal S, Canellos GP, Whang-Peng J, Gralnick HR: Blast crisis of chronic granulocytic leukemia. Morphologic variations and therapeutic implications. Am J Med 63:542–547, 1977.
2. Janossy G, Woodruff RK, Paxton A, et al.: Membrane marker and cell separation studies in Ph^1-positive leukemia. Blood 51:861–877, 1978.
3. Hong WK, Wittes RE, Hajdu ST, et al.: The evolution of mature teratoma from malignant testicular tumors. Cancer 40:2987–2992, 1977.
4. Einhorn LH, Williams SD, Mandelbaum I, Donohue JP: Surgical resection in disseminated testicular cancer following chemotherapeutic cytoreduction. Cancer 48:904–908, 1981.
5. Jones R, Hubbard SM, Osborne C, et al.: Histologic conversions in Hodgkin's lymphoma: Evolution of nodular lymphomas to diffuse lymphomas. Clin Res 26:437A, 1978.
6. DeVita VT Jr: Human models of human diseases; breast cancer and the lymphomas. Int J Radiation Oncology Biol Phys 5:1855–1867, 1979.
7. Baylin SB, Mendelsohn G: Time dependent changes in human tumors: Implications for diagnosis and clinical behaviour. Semin Oncol, 1982 (in press).
8. Research news: Tumors: A mixed bag of cells. Science 215:275–277, 1982.
9. Brereton HD, Matthews MJ, Costa J, et al.: Mixed anaplastic small-cell and squamous-cell carcinoma of the lung. Ann Intern Med 88:805–806, 1978.
10. Abeloff MD, Eggleston JC, Mendelsohn G: Changes in morphologic and biochemical characteristics of small cell carcinoma of the lung. A clinicopathologic study. Am J Med 66:757–764, 1979.
11. Matthews MJ: Effects of therapy on the morphology and behaviour of small cell carcinoma of the lung – A clinicopathologic study. In: Lung Cancer: Progress in Therapeutic Research. Muggia F, Rosenzweig M (eds). New York: Raven Press, 1979, pp 155–165.
12. Abeloff MD, Eggleston JC: Morphologic changes following therapy. In: Small Cell Lung Cancer. Greco FA, Oldham RK, Bunn PA (eds). New York: Grune and Stratton, 1981, pp 235–259.
13. Gazdar AF, Carney DN, Guccion JG, Baylin SB: Small cell carcinoma of the lung: Cellular origin and relationship to other pulmonary tumors. In: Small Cell Lung Cancer. Greco FA, Oldham RK, Bunn PA (eds). New York: Grune and Stratton, 1981, pp 145–175.
14. Fer MF, Hande KR, Oldham RK, Greco FA: Changing histology in small cell carcinoma of the lung during life. Proc Amer Soc Clin Oncol 22:504 (C–672), 1981.
15. Greco FA, Richardson RL, Snell JD, et al.: Small cell lung cancer: complete remission and improved survival. Am J Med 66:652–630, 1979.
16. Greco FA, Oldham RK: Clinical management of patients with small cell lung cancer. In: Small Cell Lung Cancer. Greco FA, Oldham RK, Bunn PA (eds). New York: Grune and Stratton, 1981, pp 353–379.
17. Gazdar AF, Zweig MH, Carney DN, et al.: Levels of creatinine kinase and its BB isoenzyme in lung cancer specimens and cultures. Cancer Res 41:2773–2777, 1981.
18. Matthews MJ, Gazdar AF: Pathology of small cell carcinoma of the lung and its subtypes. A clinico-pathologic correlation. In: Lung Cancer I. Livingston RB (ed). The Hague: Martinus Nijhoff, 1981, pp 283–306.
19. Fer MF, Sherwin SA, Oldham RK, Greco FA, Matthews MJ: Poorly differentiated lung cancer. Semin Oncol, 1982 (in press).
20. Bates M, Levison V, Hurt R, Sutton M: Treatment of oat-cell carcinoma of bronchus by preoperative radiotherapy and surgery. Lancet 1:1134–1135, 1974.
21. Larsson S, Zettergren L: Histological typing of lung cancer. Application of the World Health Organization Classification to 479 cases. Acta Path Microbiol Scan Sect A, 84:529–537, 1976.

22. Baylin SB, Mendelsohn G: Time-dependent changes in human tumors: Implications for diagnosis and clinical behaviour. Semin Oncol, 1982 (in press).
23. Auerbach O, Stout AP, Hammond CE, Garfinkel L: multiple primary bronchial carcinomas. Cancer 20:699–705, 1967.
24. Mobley DF, Martinez AJ: Two histologically different primary carcinomas of the lung. A review of the literature.
25. Martini N, Melamed MR: Multiple primary lung cancers. J Thor Cardiovasc Surg 70: 606–612, 1975.
26. Feinstein AR, Gelfman NA, Yesner R, et al.: Observer variability in the histopathologic diagnosis of lung cancer. Am Rev Resp Dis 101:671–684, 1970.
27. Stanley KE, Matthews MJ: Analysis of a pathology review of patients with lung tumors. J Natl Cancer Inst 66:989–992, 1982.
28. Rosen S, Cuttitta F, Abrams P, et al.: A monoclonal antibody (MA) which distinguishes human small cell lung cancer (SCLC) from other lung cancer types. Proc Am Assoc Cancer Res 22:303, 1981.
29. Abrams P, Rosen S, Cuttitta F: A monoclonal antibody (MA) defining an antigen expressed by non-small cell lung cancer (NSCLC), certain other human tumors, cultured skin cell lines but not normal tissues. Proc Am Soc Clin Oncol 22:373, 1981.
30. Whang-Peng J, Kao-Shan CS, Lee EC, et al.: Specific chromosome defect associated with human small-cell lung cancer: Deletion 3p (14–23). Science 215:181–182, 1982.

8. Lung Cancer Cachexia

ROWAN T. CHLEBOWSKI, DAVID HEBER, JEROME B. BLOCK

1. INTRODUCTION

Weight loss in patients with advanced lung carcinoma has been recognized clinically for many years. However, only recently has the prognostic significance of weight loss in patients with this disease been identified. In one report by Costa and co-workers [1] the incidence, timing, and severity of weight loss in a total of 479 patients with lung cancer was related to patient survival. At their initial clinical presentation, 47% of lung cancer patients had lost at least 5% of their usual body weight. The survival of these patients was significantly less than that of patients not experiencing weight loss, even when corrected for factors such as age, sex, extent of disease, cell type and performance score [1]. An analysis of 1,026 patients from the Eastern Cooperative Oncology Group revealed evidence of weight loss during the previous 6 months in 57% of small cell and 61% of non-small cell lung cancer patients [2]. In both categories of lung cancer, median survival was significantly decreased for patients experiencing antecedent weight loss prior to protocol chemotherapy: 34 weeks vs 27 weeks in small cell; 20 weeks vs 14 weeks in non-small cell. The influence of weight loss on survival in these large reports exceeds the current influence of chemotherapy on survival in non-small cell disease. Thus, weight loss at the time of clinical presentation is an important, independent factor prognostic of survival in patients with lung cancer.

2. ANOREXIA

The pathogenesis of weight loss in patients with lung carcinoma is at the present time, not completely understood. Anorexia leading to a decreased caloric intake has been recognized clinically for many years in patients with

Greco, FA (ed), Biology and Management of Lung Cancer. ISBN 0-89838-554-7.
© *1983, Martinus Nijhoff Publishers, Boston. Printed in The Netherlands.*

this disease and several hypothesis regarding its development have been proposed [3, 4, 5]. Suggested factors contributing to anorexia include: alterations of taste sensation, metabolic products such as lactate or ketones, hypothetical tumor toxins, direct effects on the appetite center and psychological influences. Alterations in taste sensation has received considerable attention. Abnormal taste sensation, in some cases associated with decreased caloric intake [6–9] has been described in cancer patients. Although some investigators report a decreased taste recognition threshold for bitter taste [9, 10], the most consistent abnormality seen is an increased taste recognition threshold for sweet substances, occurring in approximately one third of patients tested with a variety of tumors [4, 6]. The relationship among taste sensation abnormalities, the presence of cancer and the development of weight loss has been brought into question recently by observations identifying factors other than malignancy which influence these taste thresholds. For instance, although a smoking history and advancing age [11–13] have been shown to profoundly influence taste thresholds, these parameters are also associated with the development of lung cancer. In an attempt to determine the caloric importance of factors influencing taste threshold in cancer patients, we have recently evaluated taste recognition thresholds in 93 patients with malignancy including 18 patients with lung carcinoma, comparing results to 61 control patients. In cancer patients, no cases of a decreased threshold to bitter taste were detected. Thirty-eight percent of patients with cancer had an increased threshold for sweet substances, a proportion significantly greater than seen in control patients without cancer ($p < 0.01$). However, when correction using a multivariate analysis was made for smoking history and age of study patients, no difference in taste test parameters were seen between cancer patients and control patients without malignancy. In addition, we did not find an association between caloric intake, and taste test abnormalities in our cancer patient population. Although other possible mechanisms relating the presence of lung cancer to the development of anorexia have been proposed [3–5, 14], a primary role for decreased caloric intake being responsible for the development of weight loss in patients with lung cancer cannot be currently supported.

3. CALORIC AND ENERGY BALANCE

A large study has compared quantitative food intakes of 205 normal individuals to 198 ambulatory cancer patients using a 24-hour recall technique [1]. Although the caloric intake of normal males, free of cancer, significantly exceeded that for males with lung cancer (2358 kcal *vs* 1778 kcal, $p < 0.005$) essentially no difference in caloric intake between normal females and females with lung cancer was seen. Furthermore, the caloric intake for cancer patients who had lost body weight compared to those who had been able to maintain their body weight was nearly identical (1776 kcal *vs* 1780 kcal). Thus, anorexia or reduced caloric intake could not account for the weight loss experienced by these lung cancer patients. In further support of the concept that factors other than decreased caloric intake play a major role in the development of weight loss or cachexia in lung cancer patients is the failure of provision of calories alone via forced feeding [15, 16] or hyper-alimentation [17, 18] to uniformly increase lean body mass in patients with cancer. Such observations suggest that weight loss may be related to altered host metabolism brought about by the presence of malignancy.

Relatively few studies have directly evaluated energy balance in cancer patients. Basal metabolic rate determinations in cancer patients have resulted in a relatively wide range of values [19–22] with abnormally increased basal metabolic rates seen in about 35% of patients. Caloric intake and expenditure have been estimated in cancer patients and compared to results obtained in a control population group. Both decreased energy intake and increased energy expenditure were seen in the cancer patients [23]. In another study, the resting metabolic expenditure of cancer patients was determined at a defined postprandial period using a closed circuit technique with a McKesson apparatus. Resting metabolic expenditure under these circumstances was found to be abnormally high in about 50% of patients with a strong correlation between resting metabolic expenditure and weight loss and resting metabolic expenditure and serum transferrin seen [24]. These latter observations can not be directly related to the problem of lung cancer cachexia since patients with either lung cancer or metastases to the lung were specifically excluded from the latter study [24]. In summary, two studies using different methodologies support the concept that increased demands for energy are present in patients with advanced malignancy.

Changes in body composition associated with cancer cachexia have been evaluated recently using several different techniques. Watson and Sammon determined parameters of composition in cachexia resulting from both malignant disease and nonmalignant inflammatory disease using skin fold thickness and radioisotope tracer measurements [25]. The 10 male cancer patients (including 2 patients with lung carcinoma) experienced a greater degree of loss of total body fat measured by skin fold thickness changes than did patients with cachexia secondary to inflammatory disease. As a result, the calculated value for lean body mass appeared to be better conserved in the patients with weight loss and cancer than in patients with inflammatory disease and weight loss. A more detailed assessment of body composition in cancer patients with weight loss was recently reported by Cohn and co-workers [26] who used a prompt gamma neutron activation and whole body counting techniques to assess the mass and protein content of the muscle compartment. Total body water in their study was estimated with the use of tritium label. Lean body mass was calculated from their results. A total of 29 patients with malignancy and 10 normal patients were evaluated including 6 patients with lung carcinoma. The lung cancer patients had lost 6.8% of their usual body weight at the time of evaluation. The patients studied with gastrointestinal malignancy and head and neck cancer had lost nearly 20% of their usual body weight at the time of evaluation. A marked reduction of skeletal muscle tissue and protein content was seen in patients with solid tumors. Thus, the skeletal muscle compartment was a major site of the weight loss experienced by patients with solid tumors. Little change in either weight or body composition occurred in the 8 patients with hematologic malignancies. A major finding of the analysis was related to changes in the fat compartment. Although patients with lung cancer lost, on average, 25% of their body fat as compared to the control group, the relative sparing of body fat in the presence of wasting was remarkable. Even in cases of severe weight loss, lung cancer patients retain relatively large amounts of body fat. The prevalence of undernutrition in hospitalized cancer patients was recently evaluated in an 84-patient study. Using a variety of biochemical and anthropometric techniques, Nixon and co-workers [27] found the creatinine to height ratio (abnormal in 88%) to be a more sensitive index of undernutrition than anthropometrics. They concluded that protein-calorie malnutrition was commonly present in hospitalized cancer patients but was often obscured at the bedside by residual obesity.

4. ABNORMAL METABOLISM IN THE CANCER-BEARING HOST

Abnormal carbohydrate metabolism as manifest by oral glucose intolerance had been described in studies of patients with progressive weight loss and cancer for at least 60 years [28–30]. The glucose intolerance is associated with a marked resistance to administered insulin [31, 32], but the mechanism underlying this insulin resistance has not been well defined. Accelerated gluconeogenesis has been suggested as one factor contributing to the glucose intolerance of patients with carcinoma [33, 34]. Under appropriate hormonal conditions, glucose can be synthesized from substrates such as lactate and glucogenic amino acids. Glucose production from amino acids or lactate requires a significant amount of energy. Thus, if such pathways were activated inappropriately and in excess, futile cycling and net energy loss would occur. An excess substrate for gluconeogenesis can occur in cancer patients for a number of reasons. Systemic lactic acidosis has been reported by Block and others [35, 36] in patients with malignancies. However, although lactate is released into the circulation by tumor cells, lactate levels are not commonly elevated in patients with cancer. It has been estimated that the Cori cycle from glucose to lactate back to glucose may account for a 10% increase in energy expenditure in patients with cancer[18].

Amino acids released from muscle breakdown represent another potential substrate for gluconeogenesis. There is little data on plasma amino acid levels in cancer patients. In 1978, Clark, Lewis, and Waterhouse[37] studied peripheral arterial and venous blood concentrations of amino acids after an overnight fast in 4 groups of subjects: (1) malnourished cancer patients; (2) cancer patients without weight loss; (3) malnourished subjects without cancer; and (4) normal adults. Glucogenic amino acids were decreased in both malnourished cancer patients and malnourished subjects without cancer, a characteristic finding for chronic starvation. However, branched chain amino acids remained normal in cancer cachexia. The authors interpreted these findings as showing an increased rate of gluconeogenesis in patients with weight loss and cancer. Accelerated glucose turnover, determined using radiolabeled infusion techniques, has been described in a small number of patients with progressive weight loss and cancer[38–40]. Such observations suggest that futile cycling of carbohydrates by energy wasting pathways contributes to the problem of cancer cachexia[41]. We have recently demonstrated that glucose turnover shows a progressive increase when patients with cancer are evaluated serially over a several month period[30]. Gold[33] has proposed that accelerated gluconeogenesis in the host is the initial abnormality responsible for the development of cancer cachexia. If this hypothesis is correct, inhibition of the gluconeogenic pathway could provide an approach to the treatment of cancer cachexia[42].

With respect to protein metabolism, Fenninger and Mider[43] proposed in 1954 that tumors acted as nitrogen traps, siphoning protein away from the host based on data derived from studies of rats implanted with Walker 256 carcinoma. However, tumors in humans do not reach the proportions of total body weight obtained in rats, thus making such a simple trapping process an unlikely explanation for cachexia in man. Observations in man have supported the contention that synthesis of muscle proteins is generally depressed in cancer patients[44–46]. However, when whole body protein synthesis and turnover has been evaluated in a series of 7 malnourished patients with known malignancy using labeled glycine, 3 of 7 patients had marked elevations in total body protein synthesis and turnover. Protein turnover was further increased in 5 of 7 cancer patients receiving total parenteral nutrition. The mechanism underlying this accelerated protein turnover in patients with malignancy has not yet been determined[47].

As mentioned previously in a section on body composition, changes in the fat compartment are also commonly seen in patients with weight loss and cancer. Loss of body fat can occur during early stages of the cancer process when the tumor burden is not large, since Axelrod and Costa [48] have demonstrated fat loss in muscle samples obtained at the time of primary operation from patients with various tumors. With respect to the role of free fatty acids, observations suggesting both increased utilization of free fatty acids [49], and those suggesting decreased mobilization of free fatty acids in cancer patients have been reported [48]. Since liver dysfunction can be associated with elevated free fatty acids, some of the discrepancies regarding free fatty acid levels in cancer may be related to differences in liver function in various experimental groups. Investigations into hormones normally controlling lipid metabolism have demonstrated abnormalities with a decreased triiodothymidine level seen in patients with advanced cancer [48]. However, such changes also could be secondary to the decreased nutritional status seen in these patients.

In summary, changes in protein, carbohydrate, and fat metabolism have been described in patients with weight loss and lung cancer and include increased glucose production and increased muscle catabolism. Whether attempts to correct such biochemical abnormalities will alter patient weight loss or survival remain to be determined.

Derangements in the hormonal balance of patients with carcinoma and weight loss has received little systematic attention. Reduced insulin sensitivity, referred to previously, is the only major hormonal abnormality described in patients with cancer cachexia [31, 32]. Since gonadal steroids in the male promote nitrogen retention and may be important in maintaining body protein stores [50] we investigated gonadal hormonal function prior to chemotherapy in men with advanced malignancy. Forty-four adult male patients with histologically proven metastatic cancer including 10 patients with lung carcinoma were studied. Serum LH, βHCG, and total testosterone were measured by specific radioimmunoassay and the percent free testosterone was calculated. These values were compared to the normal values determined in our laboratory of 21 age-matched adult males without cancer. In 43% of patients with cancer, serum testosterone was less than the lower limit of normal; free testosterone in the cancer patients was below the control range in 29 cases (66%). Four patterns of serum testosterone and LH were seen in patients with cancer: (1) normal testosterone and normal LH in 12 cases; (2) normal testosterone and high LH in 13 cases, consistent with early primary hypogonadism; (3) low testosterone and high LH in 10 cases, consistent with frank primary hypogonadism; and (4) low testosterone and low/normal LH in 9 cases, consistent with secondary hypogonadism. Significantly decreased ideal body weight was found in the group with low testosterone and low or normal LH levels. Table 1 relates ideal body weight with

Table 1. Relationship among testosterone level, LH, and percent ideal body weight in patients with metastatic carcinoma.

Group	Patient number	Testosterone level	LH	Percent ideal body weight
1	12	normal[a]	normal[a]	96±4
2	13	normal	high	93±3
3	10	low	high	87±3
4	9	low	normal or low	84±3[b]

[a] Compared to 21 age-matched controls without cancer.
[b] Significantly different ($p<0.05$) compared to Group 1.

androgen levels in this population. Thus, decreased gonadal hormone secretion is seen in adult males with advanced cancer and malnutrition, even prior to chemotherapy treatment. The observed hypogonadism may be a factor contributing to the development of the protein-calorie malnutrition commonly seen in patients with cancer. Prospective studies of androgen replacement in such patients will be required, however, to assess this possibility [51].

As we have seen, many of the metabolic and hormonal derangements said to occur in lung cancer patients with weight loss have been described as isolated findings in patients studied in different institutions. To investigate the relationship among several of these metabolic parameters we have recently evaluated a series of patients with non-small cell lung cancer during a metabolic ward admission and compared the results to those obtained from a group of chronic lung disease patients without cancer evaluated in a similar fashion [52]. Patients with lung cancer were studied either before ($n = 6$) or after ($n = 6$) the development of significant weight loss from ideal body weight (Table 2). Caloric intake by history, body surface area, and basal metabolic rate determinations were not significantly different between the three groups. The calculated basal energy expenditure was somewhat lower in the malnourished lung cancer group, and as a result, the ratio of measured basal metabolic rate to calculated basal energy expenditure was higher in the malnourished cancer patient group, but not significantly so. The 5-day period of hospitalization included: protein turnover using the continuous infusion of C^{14} lysine; glucose turnover using continuous infusion of glucose 6H3; glucose tolerance using standard oral glucose tolerance testing; nitrogen balance determination and hormonal status assessment. Lung cancer patients with and without malnutrition and controls excreted similar quantities of nitrogen. Total body protein turnover was significantly increased ($p<0.05$) in malnourished cancer patients compared

Table 2. Glucose and protein metabolism in patients with non-small cell lung cancer studied either before or after the development of weight loss.[c]

Group	N	Age	% Ideal body weight	Triceps skin fold (mm)	Glucose production (mg/kg/min)[a]	3-methyl-histidine excretion (μmole/ g creat/ 24 hr)[b]
Control	6	57 ± 4	106 ± 3	27 ± 4	2.0 ± 0.1	71 ± 10
Normal weight cancer	6	63 ± 3	103 ± 4	20 ± 3	2.6 ± 0.1^{d}	105 ± 17^{d}
Malnourished cancer	6	64 ± 4	80 ± 2^{d}	11 ± 2^{d}	2.9 ± 0.2^{d}	111 ± 13^{d}

[a] Determined by a constant infusion of 6-^{3}H-glucose in the fasting state.
[b] Determined by a constant infusion of ^{14}C-lysine in the fasting state on day 5 of constant nitrogen and caloric intake.
[c] Published in part in Cancer Res 42:4815, 1982.
[d] Difference from control group is significantly different ($p<0.05$).

to either well-nourished cancer patients or controls. Muscle catabolism was determined by quantitating urinary ^{3}methylhistidine-creatinine excretion ratios and was increased in both well-nourished and normal weight cancer patients compared to controls. Glucose production rates were also increased in both malnourished and normal weight cancer patients compared to controls (Table 2). Thus, both increased glucose production and increased muscle catabolism were evident metabolic abnormalities in patients with non-small cell lung cancer prior to the development of malnutrition. Identification of these metabolic abnormalities as an integral part of the non-small cell lung cancer disease process permits further evaluation of therapies designed to prevent cancer cachexia.

We have expanded these observations of abnormal glucose metabolism in a larger series of 25 patients with a variety of metastatic cancers [30]. During their initial evaluation, fasting blood sugar was less than 110 mg % in 22 of 25 cancer patients evaluated, and abnormal glucose tolerance was frequently seen. At 2 hours following glucose ingestion, glucose was 173 ± 13 mg % with an associated insulin of 65 ± 12 I units/ml. In this population, growth hormone and cortisol were normal in all cases and only 3 patients had abnormal fasting glucagon values. Six patients had repeat evaluations of glucose turnover and oral glucose tolerance tests 1 month after initial evaluation. Glucose tolerance remained abnormal while glucose turnover increased from 2.9 ± 0.2 mg/kg/minute to 3.4 ± 0.2 mg/kg/minute.

Seven patients with non-small cell lung cancer were among the 25 evaluated. We concluded from these serial observations that malnutrition in cancer patients is associated with progressive abnormalities in glucose production. The progressive abnormality in glucose turnover represents a possible point of therapeutic intervention in patients with cancer cachexia.

Consideration of the gluconeogenic pathway shows it to be amenable to therapeutic intervention at the phosphoenol-pyruvate carboxykinase (PEPCK) reaction, the enzymatic step which catalyzes the conversion of oxaloacetate acid to phosphoenol-pyruvate (PEP). The compound hydrazine sulfate has been found to be a noncompetitive inhibitor of PEPCK [33], with resultant inhibition of *in vitro* gluconeogenesis in a number of animal systems [53, 54]. This compound is, in addition, an inhibitor of *in vivo* growth of a number of transplantable animal tumors [55], as well as being closely related structurally to the recognized cytotoxic agent methylhydrazine (procarbazine). Hydrazine sulfate has had preliminary evaluation as an anti-cachexia and cytotoxic agent both in this country [56] as well as in Russia [57] with some beneficial effects reported. However, not all studies of hydrazine sulfate have shown unequivocal benefit [58, 59]; the studies with negative results were not designed to assess either subjective improvement or influence on cancer cachexia. No study, either in man or animal model system, has attempted to correlate inhibition of the gluconeogenic pathway with anti-cachexia effects in the same subjects. A major difficulty in the past complicating interpretation of clinical hydrazine trials has been study designs which did not evaluate changes in metabolic parameters. In addition, the selection of therapeutic endpoints have been inappropriate, either using solely subjective criteria or assessing only antitumor effect. As a result, both the positive [56, 57] and negative [58, 59] clinical trials have not given incontrovertable results. Thus, well-designed studies which can evaluate antitumor response, quantitative parameters of cancer cachexia, and subjective symptomatology and correlate such findings with alterations in glucose turnover are needed to accurately define the role of hydrazine sulfate in cancer cachexia. To address this question we have initiated at the Harbor-UCLA Medical Center, a randomized, double-blind, placebo-controlled trial to evaluate the influence of hydrazine sulfate on abnormal carbohydrate metabolism in patients with weight loss and cancer. Glucose tolerance and total body glucose turnover will be determined both before and after one month of therapy with either hydrazine sulfate or a placebo compound. The results of this trial should define whether or not hydrazine sulfate influences the accelerated glucose production seen in patients with malignancy.

5. THERAPEUTIC NUTRITIONAL INTERVENTIONS

While the influence of weight loss on survival in lung cancer patients is clear, the ability of existing methods of nutritional intervention to prevent or reverse this unfavorable outcome is not established. In severe cases of malnutrition, dietary supplements alone may be inadequate because of the malabsorption, anorexia, and gastrointestinal symptoms associated with malnourished state. Several early trials attempted to reverse the anorexia cachexia syndrome in cancer patients with forced feeding, but had mixed results [15, 16]. Experience with currently available enteral supplements has been utilized with some success in several medical [60] and surgical [61] patient populations. However, the successful use of the enteral route in providing nutritional support to these groups may not be directly applicable to the unique situation of cancer patients. In fact, only limited information on the use of tube feedings in a small number of cancer patients has been published [62]. We have recently evaluated an inexpensive blenderized tube feeding formula in cachectic patients with a variety of malignancies. Progressive weight loss was interrupted in 7 of 9 patients after 2 weeks of therapy but clinical outcome was not changed [63]. Nixon and co-workers [64] have compared intravenous central to enteral hyperalimentation in a nonrandomized study in which serial anthropometrics and biochemical parameters were used to assess changes in lean body mass. Such results suggest comparable efficacy for enteral and parenteral routes of administration [40, 65]. However, nutritional supplementation was less successful in cancer patients compared to noncancer patients as measured by standard indexes. One trial has prospectively evaluated enteral support in lung cancer patients with moderate malnutrition who were treated with chemotherapy [66]. In addition to chemotherapy, routine nutrition was compared to nasogastric administration of 3,000 calories per day. A protective effect of enteral support on hematopoietic toxicity of chemotherapy was reported. Further studies will be needed to more precisely define the role of continuous enteral supplementation in patients with lung cancer cachexia.

The introduction of total parenteral nutrition (TPN) has permitted the physician to provide nutritional support without utilizing the gastrointestinal tract [67]. Early clinical experience in nonrandomized trials have suggested TPN to be beneficial in converting skin tests and decreasing toxic effects associated with chemotherapeutic regimens [67]. In addition, the development of Hickman [68] and Broviac [69] catheters has simplified the long-term use of TPN. Despite the well-documented ability of TPN to increase weight of cancer patients, the results of randomized trials where TPN was the treatment variable have been less encouraging with respect to improving clinical outcome [70, 71].

There is general agreement that nutritional intervention is indicated in cancer patients in whom severe malnutrition precludes administration of potentially efficacious therapy. However, even in a population of patients with a wasting disease like lung cancer, such individuals constitute a distinct minority of cases. The role of nutritional support in the care of the majority of lung cancer patients has not yet been clearly defined. The problems inherent in attempting to identify a subpopulation of lung cancer patients who might benefit from nutritional support has been recently reviewed [72]. At the present time only a limited number of outcome-oriented randomized studies involving parenteral nutritional support have been reported for patients with lung carcinoma. In a study conducted at M.D. Anderson Hospital, 65 patients with extensive adenocarcinoma of the lung were randomized to receive 4-drug intensive chemotherapy with or without intravenous hyperalimentation beginning 10 days prior to chemotherapy and continuing through the first course for a median of 35 days. Although survival was longer in patients with less than 6% pretreatment weight loss, there was no difference in survival among the three nutritional treatment groups. In addition, only minimal protection from chemotherapy induced gastrointestinal and hematological toxic effects by intravenous hyperalimentation was described. The early analyses of this study suggested significant protection from myelosuppression in patients receiving pre-chemotherapy intravenous hyperalimentation [73] but these observations were not confirmed in the final analysis [74]. Patients receiving nutritional support did demonstrate increased body weight during the first two courses of chemotherapy compared to patients not receiving parenteral nutritional support. However, this alteration in body weight did not translate into improved survival or decreased toxicity in this adenocarcinoma patient population. In a separate study involving patients with small cell lung cancer, Valdivieso and coworkers [75] have treated 49 patients with 4-drug chemotherapy including VP-16, doxorubicin, vincristine, and cyclophosphamide with or without intravenous hyperalimentation throughout the first two courses of in-patient therapy. The extreme myelosuppression of this regimen with a median neutrophil count of 0 was not influenced by nutritional support. Intravenous hyperalimentation also did not influence significantly other hematologic, gastrointestinal or infectious morbidity of this intensive 4-drug chemotherapy regimen. Preservation of weight and improved skin reactivity to skin antigens was observed with nutritional intervention. Although a higher complete remission rate was seen for patients receiving intravenous hyperalimentation, only tentative conclusions regarding efficacy can be drawn from this preliminary report. A third randomized trial of TPN by the same group, demonstrates somewhat more favorable results in patients with epidermoid cell carcinoma [76]. The addition of TPN (35 kcal/kg of patient body weight/day) for 10 days prior to and 21 days following the first course of chemoimmunotherapy with *C. parvum,* isophosphamide and doxorubicin resulted in significantly decreased nausea and myelosuppression for 13 TPN patients compared to 13 not receiving TPN. The TPN patients also had a suggestion of therapeutic benefit (31% response *vs* 7%) but this difference was not significant. Compared to the intensive attempts at nutritional support administered in the preceding three studies, Serrou and co-workers [77] have evaluated the efficacy of a much less intensive peripheral intravenous nutrition program in lung cancer patients of two histological types. Patients in both trials were randomly allocated to receive nutritional support or not in the form of peripheral intravenous hyperalimentation. Each patient received only 1500 kcal per day. All patients studied had histologically diagnosed small cell bronchial carcinoma or epidermoid carcinoma. Patients with small cell tumors received combination chemotherapy including doxorubicin, VP-16, and vincristine and patients received between 8 and 20 days of nutritional support. A similar nutritional support program was involved for patients with epidermoid tumors who received chemoimmunotherapy followed by radiotherapy. Therapy consisted of doxorubicin, vincristine, CCNU, 5-fluorouracil, and BCG. For patients with small cell carcinoma there was no difference between the two groups in either patient weight or survival at 24 months. Bone marrow toxicity and gastrointestinal toxicity were also similar in the two groups. For patients with epidermoid tumors, quite different results were seen. There was a significant ($p < 0.001$) increase in survival for the group receiving peripheral intravenous nutrition associated with radiochemoimmunotherapy: 6-month survival of 60% for the group receiving radiotherapy alone *vs* 77% for the group receiving radiochemoimmunotherapy associated with peripheral intravenous nutrition. This intriguing preliminary result suggests that the administration of a relatively limited number of calories during the course of a defined treatment program can result in improved survival in patients with epidermoid lung cancer. Detailed metabolic and nutritional evaluations of such patients will be required to address the question of how the administration of a relatively limited number of additional calories for a short period of treatment can result in increased survival. In summary, the currently available randomized clinical trials involving parenteral nutrition in the treatment of patients with advanced lung cancer do not support the routine use of this modality of therapy at the present time. Two studies, from the United States [76] and France [77] have observed interesting preliminary results in squamous cell carcinoma patients receiving chemoimmunotherapy and nutritional support. Randomized studies involving total parenteral nutrition as an adjunct to chemotherapy in other disease types have also reported similar equivocal findings [70, 72]. At present, the clinical situation where nutritional intervention has received the most support is in the preoperative parenteral feeding given to patients with gastrointestinal malignancies [78]. No studies on the preoperative nutritional support of patients with lung carcinoma have yet been reported. Based on the results of the randomized trials in lung cancer patients, a study of preoperative nutritional support of patients with squamous cell carcinoma and weight loss would be most interesting. The results of currently available randomized trials of nutritional support in lung cancer patients are summarized in Table 3.

6. SUMMARY

In summary, we may conclude that weight loss in the patient with lung cancer is associated with a poor prognosis for long-term survival [1, 80]. Abnormalities of protein, carbohydrate, and fat metabolism have been defined in patients with cancer cachexia and appear to represent derange-

Table 3. Results of prospective, randomized trials in the use of parenteral nutritional support in advanced lung cancer.

Author (reference)	Patient number	Lung carcinoma cell type	Therapy	Effect of parenteral nutrition *versus* control results
Lanzotti [79] (abstract)	33	non-small cell	chemo	decrease in WBC nadir on TPN, no difference in response or survival
Valdivieso [75] (abstract)	30	small cell	chemo	increase (not significant) in complete responses on TPN
Serrou [77]	40	small cell	chemo	no difference in response or toxicity on PIN
Jordan [74]	65	adenocarcinoma	chemo	no difference in response or toxicity on TPN
Issell [26]	26	squamous cell	chemo, immuno	decrease in nausea and WBC nadir on TPN; increase (not significant) in partial response rate on TPN
Serrou [77]	70	squamous cell	chemo, immuno, radiation	significant increase in survival on PIN

TPN = Total parenteral nutrition.
PIN = Peripheral intravenous nutrition.

ments in host metabolism induced by the cancer. While the impact of weight loss on survival in lung cancer is evident, the ability of existing methods of nutritional intervention including enteral and total parenteral nutrition to prevent, reverse, or treat malnutrition in this patient population remains to be established. A number of hypotheses have been developed to account for rapid weight loss in lung cancer patients despite the administration of apparently adequate calories [81]. These include excess energy consumption by the tumor, hormonal imbalances, and excess futile cycling of carbohydrates by the host leading to energy wasting. The consensus view at the present time is that the cancer somehow deranges host metabolism. A large number of investigations are currently aimed at elucidating the etiology of cancer cachexia in lung cancer patients as well as the efficacy of new approaches to therapeutic intervention.

ACKNOWLEDGMENT

Some of the work reported received support from NIH Grant CA 26563 and the General Clinical Research Center Grant RR-00425 as well as from the American Cancer Society Grant MG 3965.

REFERENCES

1. Costa G, Lane WW, Vincent RG, Siebold JA, Aragon M, Bewley PT: Weight loss and cachexia in lung cancer. Nutrition and Cancer 2:98–103, 1981.
2. DeWys WD, Begg C, Lavin PT, et al.: Prognostic effect of weight loss prior to chemotherapy in cancer patients. Am J Med 69:491–498, 1980.
3. Bernstein IL: Physiological and psychological mechanisms of cancer anorexia. Cancer Res (suppl) 42:715s–720s, 1982.
4. DeWys WD: Anorexia as a general effect of cancer. Cancer 43:2013–2019, 1979.
5. Theologides A: Anorexia in cancer: another speculation on its pathogenesis: Nutrition and Cancer 2:133–135, 1981.
6. DeWys WD, Walters K: Abnormalities of taste sensation in cancer patients. Cancer 36:1888–1896, 1975.
7. DeWys WD: Taste abnormalities and caloric intake in cancer patients: a review. J Human Nutr 32:447–453, 1978.
8. Carson JAS, Gormican A: Taste acquity and food attitudes of selected patients with cancer. J Am Diet Assoc 70:361–364, 1977.
9. Williams LR, Cohen MH: Altered taste thresholds in lung cancer. Am J Clin Nutr 31:122–125, 1978.
10. Hall JC, Staniland JR, Giles I: Altered taste thresholds in gastrointestinal cancer. Clinical Oncology 6:137–142, 1980.
11. Conger AD, Wells MA: Radiation and aging effects on taste structure and function. Radiation Res 37:31–38, 1969.
12. Kaplan AR: The effect of cigarette smoking on malnutrition and digestion. Gastroenterology 61:208, 1963.

13. Henkin R: Taste loss in aging. In: The Biomedical Role of Trace Elements in Aging. Davis HJ, Neithmeimer R, St Petersburg R (eds). Eckerd College Gerontology Center, 1976, pp 221–236.

14. Barai B, DeWys W: Assay for presence of anorectic substance in urine of cancer patients. Proc Amer Assoc Can Res 21:378, 1980.

15. Pareira MD, Conrad EJ, Hicks W, Elman R: Clinical response and changes in nitrogen balance, body weight, plasma proteins, and hemoglobin following tube feeding in cancer cachexia. Cancer 8:803–808, 1955.

16. Terepka AR, Waterhouse C: Metabolic observations during forced feeding of patients with cancer. Am J Med 20:225–238, 1956.

17. Rickard KA, Kirsey A, Baehner RL, et al.: Nutritional management of children with advanced cancer: effectiveness of enteral and parenteral nutrition. Fed Proc 38:865, 1979.

18. Young VR: Energy metabolism and requirements in the cancer patient. Cancer Res 37:2336–2341, 1977.

19. Silver S, Poroto P, Crohn EB: Hypermetabolic states without hyperthyroidism. Arch Intern Med 85:479–482, 1950.

20. Waterhouse C: How tumors affect host metabolism. Ann NY Acad Sci 230:86–93, 1974.

21. Waterhouse CL, Fenninger LD, Kentmann EH: Nitrogen exchange and caloric expenditure in patients with malignant neoplasm. Cancer 4:500–514, 1951.

22. Watkin DM: Nitrogen balance as affected by neoplastic disease and its therapy. Am J Clin Nutr 9:446–460, 1961.

23. Warnold I, Lundholm K, Schersten T: Energy balance and body composition in cancer patients. Cancer Res 38:1801–1807, 1978.

24. Bozzetti F, Pagnoni AM, Vecchio MD: Excessive caloric expenditures as a cause of malnutrition in patients with cancer. Surg Gyn Obstet 150: 229–234, 1980.

25. Watson WS, Sammon AM: Body composition in cachexia resulting from malignant and non-malignant disease. Cancer 46:2041–2046, 1981.

26. Cohn SH, Gartenhaus W, Sawitsky A, Rai K, Zanzi I, Vaswani A, Ellis KJ, Vartsky D: Compartmental body composition of cancer patients by measurement of total body nitrogen, potassium, and water. Metabolism 30:22–229, 1981.

27. Nixon DW, Heymsfield SB, Cohen AE, Kutner MH, Ansley J, Lawson DH, Rudman D: Protein-calorie undernutrition in hospitalized cancer patients. Am J Med 68:683–690, 1980.

28. Rohdenberg GL, Bernhard A, Krehbiel O: Sugar tolerance in cancer. JAMA 72:1528–1529, 1919.

29. Marks PA, Bishop JS: The glucose metabolism of patients with malignant disease and of normal subjects as studied by means of an intravenous glucose tolerance test. J Clin Invest 36:254–264, 1957.

30. Chlebowski RT, Heber D, Block JB: Serial assessment of glucose metabolism in patients with cancer cachexia. Clin Res 30:69A, 1982.

31. Bishop JS, Marks PA: Studies on carbohydrate metabolism in patients with neoplastic disease II. Response to insulin administration. J Clin Invest 38:688–672, 1959.

32. Schein P, Kisner D, Haller D, Blecher M, Hamosh M: Cachexia of malignancy: potential role of insulin in nutritional management. Cancer 43:2070–2076, 1979.

33. Gold J: Cancer cachexia and gluconeogenesis. Ann NY Acad Sci 230:103–110, 1975.

34. Costa G: Cachexia, the metabolic component of neoplastic disease Cancer Res 37: 2327–2335, 1977.

35. Block JB: Lactic acidosis in malignancy and observation on its possible pathogenesis. Ann NY Acad Sci 230:94–102, 1974.

36. Field M, Block JB, Leven R, Rall DP: The significance of elevations of blood lactate in

patients with neoplastic and other proliferative disorders. Am J Med 40:528–547, 1966.

37. Clark EF, Lewis AM, Waterhouse C: Peripheral amino acid levels in patients with cancer. Cancer 42:2909–2913, 1978.
38. Holroyde CP, Gabuzda TG, Putnam RC, Paul P, Reinchard GA: Altered metabolism in metastatic carcinoma. Cancer Res 35:3710–3714, 1978.
39. Reichard GA, Joury NF, Hochella NJ, et al.: Quantitative estimation of the Cori cycle in the human. J Biol Chem 238:495–501, 1963.
40. Burt ME, Gorschboth CM, Brennan MF: A controlled, prospective, randomized trial evaluating metabolic effects of enteral and parenteral nutrition in the cancer patient. Cancer 49:1092–1105, 1982.
41. Stein TP: Cachexia, gluconeogenesis and progressive weight loss in cancer patients. J Theor Biol 73:51–59, 1978.
42. Theologides A: Cancer cachexia. Cancer 43:2004–2012, 1979.
43. Fenninger LD, Mider GB: Energy and nitrogen metabolism in cancer. Adv Cancer Res 2:229, 1954.
44. Lundholm K, Bylund AC, Holm J, Scherstein T: Skeletal muscle metabolism in patients with malignant tumor. Eur J Cancer 12:465–471, 1976.
45. Lundholm K, Holm G, Schersten T: Insulin resistance in patients with cancer. Cancer Res 38:4665–4670, 1978.
46. Levin L, Gevers W: Metabolic alterations in cancer. South African Medical Journal 59:553–555, 1981.
47. Norton JA, Stein TP, Brennan MF: Whole body protein synthesis and turnover in normal man and malnourished patients with and without known cancer. Ann Surg 194:123–128, 1981.
48. Axelrod L, Costa G: The contribution of fat loss to weight loss in cancer. Nutr Cancer 2:81–83, 1980.
49. Waterhouse C, Kemperman J: Carbohydrate metabolism in subjects with cancer. Cancer Res 31:1273–1278, 1971.
50. Wilson JD, Griffin JE: The use and misuse of androgens. Metabolism 29:1278–1294, 1980.
51. Chlebowski RT, Heber D: Hypogonadism in male patients with metastatic cancer prior to chemotherapy. Cancer Res 42:2495–2498, 1982.
52. Heber D, Chlebowski RT, Ishibashi DE, Herrold JN, Block JB: Metabolic abnormalities in lung cancer patients. Cancer Res 42:4815–4819, 1982.
53. Ray PD, Hanson RL, Lardy HA: Inhibition by hydrazine of gluconeogenesis in the rat. J Biol Chem 245:690–696, 1970.
54. Fortney SR, Clark DA, Stein EJ: Inhibition of gluconeogenesis by hydrazine administration in rats. J Pharmacol Exp Ther 156:277–284, 1972.
55. Gold J: Inhibition by hydrazine sulfate and various hydrazines of in vivo growth of Walker 256 intramuscular carcinoma, B-16 melanoma, Murphy-Stern lymphosarcoma and L-1210 leukemia. Oncology 27:69–80, 1973.
56. Gold J: Use of hydrazine sulfate in terminal and preterminal cancer patients. Oncology 32:1–10, 1975.
57. Gershanovich ML, Danova LA, Ivin BA, Filov VA: Results of clinical study of antitumor action of hydrazine sulfate. Nutr and Cancer 3:7–12, 1982.
58. Spremulli E, Wampler GL, Regelson W: Clinical study of hydrazine sulfate in advanced cancer patients. Cancer Chemother Pharm 3:121–124, 1979.
59. Lerner HJ, Regelson W: Clinical trial of hydrazine sulfate in solid tumors. Cancer Treat Rep 60:959–960, 1976.

60. Heymsfield SB, Bethel RA, Ansley JD, et al.: Enteral hyperalimentation: an alternative to central venous hyperalimentation. Ann Int Med 90: 63–72, 1979.

61. Kaminski MU: Enteral hyperalimentation. Surg Gyn Obst 143:12–21, 1976.

62. Loh KK, Inasmasu MS, Melish S, et al.: Enteral hyperalimentation in the treatment of malnourished cancer patients. Proc Am Assoc Cancer Res 20:301, 1979.

63. Block JB, Chlebowski RT, Herrold J: Continuous enteric alimentation with a blenderized formular in cancer cachexia. Clin Onco 7:93–98, 1981.

64. Nixon DW, Lawson DH, Dutner M, et al.: Hyperalimentation of the cancer patients with protein-calorie undernutrition. Cancer Res 41:2038–2045, 1981.

65. Nixon DW: Hyperalimentation in the undernourished cancer patient. Cancer Res (suppl) 42:727s–728s, 1982.

66. Lipschitz DA, Mitchell CO: Enteral hyperalimentation and hematopoietic toxicity caused by chemotherapy of small cell lung cancer. JPEN 4:593, 1980.

67. Copeland EM, Macfayder BV, Dudrick SJ: Effect of hyperalimentation on established delayed hypersensitivity in the cancer patients. Ann Surg 184: 60–64, 1976.

68. Hickman RD, Buckner CD, Clift RA, et al.: A modified right atrial cathether for access to the venous system in marrow transplant recipients. Surg Gynecol Obstet 148:872–875, 1979.

69. Broviac JW, Cole JJ, Scribner BH: A silicone rubber atrial catheter for prolonged parenteral alimentation. Surg Gynecol Obstet 136:602–607, 1974.

70. Brennan MF. Total parenteral nutrition in the cancer patient. N Engl J Med 305:375–382, 1981.

71. Brennan MF, Copeland EM: Panel report on nutritional assessment and prechemotherapy hyperalimentation in adenocarcinoma of the lung. Proc Am Assoc Cancer Res 20:412, 1979.

72. Levine AS, Brennan MF, Ramu A, et al.: Controlled clinical trials of nutritional intervention as an adjacent to chemotherapy with a comment on nutrition and drug resistance. Cancer Res (suppl) 42:774s–781s, 1982.

73. Jordan WM, Valdivieso M, Freeman M, et al.: Importance of nutritional assessment and prechemotherapy hyperalimentation in adenocarcinoma of the lung. Proc Am Assoc Cancer Res 20:412, 1979.

74. Jordan WM, Valdivieso M, Frankmann C, Gillespie M, Issell BF, Bodey GP, Freireich EJ: Treatment of advanced adenocarcinoma of the lung with ftorafur, doxorubicin, cyclophosphamide, and cis-platin (FACP) and intensive IV hyperalimentation. Cancer Treat Rep 65:197–206, 1981.

75. Valdivieso M, Bodey G, Barkley T, Benjamin R, Mountain C: Randomized evaluation of intravenous hyperalimentation during intensive chemotherapy for small cell lung cancer. Proc Am Assoc Clin Oncol 21:C-560, 1980.

76. Issell BF, Valdivieso M, Zaren HA, et al.: Protection against chemotherapy toxicity by IV hyperalimentation. Cancer Treat Rep 62:1139–1143, 1978.

77. Serrou B, Cupissol D, Favier F, Michel FB: Opposite results in two randomized trials evaluating the adjunct value of peripheral intravenous nutrition in lung cancer patients. In: Adjuvant Therapy of Cancer III. Salmon SE, Jones SE (eds). New York: Grune and Stratton, 1981, pp 255–261.

78. Muller JM, Dienst C, Brenner U, Pichlmaier H: Preoperative parenteral feeding in patients with gastrointestinal carcinoma. Lancet 1:68–71, 1982.

79. Lanzotti V, Copeland E, Bhuchar V, Wesley M, Corriere J, Dudrick S: A randomized trial of total parenteral nutrition (TPN) with chemotherapy for non-oat cell lung cancer. Proc Am Assoc Can Res 21:377, 1980.

80. Lanzotti VJ, Thomas DR, Boyle LD, et al.: Survival with inoperable lung cancer: an inte-

142

gration of prognostic variables based on simple clinical criteria. Cancer 33:303–313, 1977.

81. DeWys W: Pathophysiology of cancer cachexia: current understanding and areas for future research. Cancer Res (suppl) 42:721s–726s, 1982.

9. The Neurophysins and Small Cell Lung Cancer

WILLIAM G. NORTH, L. HERBERT MAURER and JOSEPH F. O'DONNELL

1. INTRODUCTION

Neurophysins are single chain proteins of about 10,000 daltons in size that are normally produced by neurons in the hypothalamus. These proteins are rich in cysteine, glycine, and glutamic acid, and all of those so-far studied have an N-terminal alanine. Most of the neurons that produce neurophysins are located in the supraoptic and paraventricular nuclei of the anterior hypothalamus. Two other well-characterized products of these neurons are the hormones oxytocin and vasopressin (antidiuretic hormone, ADH).

2. BIOSYNTHESIS OF NEUROPHYSINS BY HYPOTHALAMIC NEURONS

The neurophysins (NPs), oxytocin (OT) and vasopressin (VP) are initially translated as larger precursors on ribosomes [1–6]. These precursors are then packaged into neurosecretory granules (NSG) in the Golgi apparatus of neurons and transported along axons, most of which terminate in the neural lobe. The NSG are about 160 nm in diameter. During passage from perikarya to axonal terminals, the precursors within the granules become transformed into peptide hormones and neurophysins by cleavage of specific peptide bonds [4, 5, 7]. It is now becoming clear that there are specific neurons that produce VP and one type of NP, and specific neurons that produce OT and another type of NP. We have named the neurophysin of vasopressinergic neurons, vasopressin-associated neurophysin (VP-NP), and the neurophysin of oxytocinergic neurons, oxytocin-associated neurophysin (OT-NP). In this scheme, human neurophysins (HNPs) are abbreviated VP-HNP and OT-HNP, respectively, while rat neurophysins (RNPs) become VP-RNP and OT-RNP. For human neurophysins, VP-HNP is synonymous with nicotine-stimulated neurophysin, and OT-HNP is synonymous with

Greco, FA (ed), Biology and Management of Lung Cancer. ISBN 0-89838-554-7.
© 1983, Martinus Nijhoff Publishers, Boston. Printed in The Netherlands.

estrogen-stimulated neurophysin, in the nomenclature earlier introduced by Robinson [8, 9].

The inseparable nature of the hormones and the neurophysins was first clearly seen in the Brattleboro rat, a remarkable animal model for inherited hypothalamic diabetes insipidus. These animals were first bred at Dartmouth by Valtin and Sokol and have recently been the subject of an international meeting [10]. Further support for adopting a hormone designation for neurophysins has come from Land and co-workers [7] who have now shown definitively that each hormone and the neurophysin with which it is associated share a common precursor.

Much of the information about the biosynthesis of VP, OT and NPs has resulted from pulse-chase studies which measured the incorporation of radiolabelled amino acids into proteins and peptides [1–3, 11]. Gainer and co-workers centered on identifying possible precursors of the neurophysins in the rat using an antiserum that did not discriminate between the two rat neurophysins, and were able to isolate molecules of 20,000 and 15,000 daltons that appeared to be precursors [3]. Precursor forms for neurophysins have also been demonstrated by cell-free translation with mRNA from bovine hypothalamus [12–14] and from rat hypothalamus [15]. Translation performed in the presence of microsomal membranes was found to convert a possible precursor form of vasopressin-associated bovine neurophysin (VP-BNP) of 21,000 daltons to a glycosylated 23,000 dalton product. These observations led Schmale and Richter [13] to conclude that the precursor of VP-NP and VP is normally glycosylated, and such a conclusion was in agreement with the data of Russell and co-workers [16] who were able to show that ^{3}H-fucose was incorporated into the neurophysin precursor associated with vasopressinergic neurons. On the other hand, the precursor of OT-NP and OT does not appear to be glycosylated [13, 14, 17], and has a molecular size between 15,000 and 18,000 daltons [13–15]. The mRNA sequence encoding a common precursor to VP-BNP and VP has now been determined, and this has been used to deduce the amino acid sequence for the precursor. The basic structure of this precursor is illustrated in Figure 1.

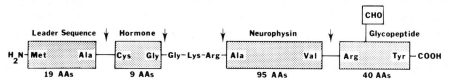

Figure 1. A schematic representation of the precursor structure for vasopressin and VP-BNP deduced by Land and co-workers showing the bonds which must ultimately be cleaved, in order to liberate free hormone and neurophysin. At least three types of enzymes seem to be required to explain the products formed, and one of these is an acid proteinase with α-chymotryptic specificity.

The precursor comprises 166 amino acids arranged in the following manner: a 19 amino acid signal peptide at the amino terminus is attached through an Ala-Cys bond to the sequence representing VP; this is followed by a sequence -Gly-Lys-Arg- and then the sequence of the NP; a 40 amino acid residue glycopeptide is attached at the carboxyl end of the NP. It is likely the common precursor to OT-NP and OT will have a similar sequence. Now that sequence information is available on the 166 amino acid precursor for VP-BNP and VP, there is a need to explain the nature of other putative precursors of larger molecular size which have been identified in extracts of hypothalamus and neural lobe [18–20]. One prominent form has a molecular weight apparent of 28,000–35,000 [18].

The generation of hormones and neurophysins occurs in the neurosecretory granules (NSG). The events involved in these transformations might therefore be interpreted from known characteristics of the granules and their components. Cannata and Morris [21] proposed that under physiological conditions the pH inside the NSG of the neural lobe is in the vicinity of 5, because they found that these NSG were most stable to fixation at this pH. Besides this, when neurophysins and hormones are generated from their common precursors they form noncovalent complexes, and the view of an intragranular pH of 5 was consistent with known characteristics of these complexes because they are stable and least-soluble in the pH range 5–6. Russell and co-workers [22] have, in fact, recently measured the pH within NSG using a dye-method and confirmed that intragranular pH is about pH 5.3. The electron microscopic studies of Morris [23] and the studies performed by us on the subcellular localization of neurophysins and hormones by RIA [24] have demonstrated that most of the neurophysins and hormones in the neural terminals of the neural lobe are located within NSG, and indicate that release of each NP and hormone is associated with the loss of the entire granule contents by exocytosis. The hormone content of each granule has been calculated to be about 10^5 molecules, and the intragranular molarity of each hormone (and neurophysin) has been estimated as being greater than $0.1\,M$ [23, 25]. It might, therefore, be inferred that granules when first formed in the neurons of the hypothalamus are each packaged with about 10^5 molecules of prohormones at a concentration of $>0.1\,M$. This high concentration of substrate for proteolysis (i.e., the prohormone) could mean that the rate of conversion to the products of proteolysis (i.e., neurophysins and hormones) is largely independent of substrate concentration.

We have used plasma values of VP-$\underline{R}$NP and OT-$\underline{R}$NP, their half-lives in the circulation, and their volumes of distribution to arrive at an estimate of their rates of production/release from the hypothalamo-neurohypophysial system of the rat [23, 26]. These studies were performed in the conscious rat and the relationship used in these calculations was based on the equation:

$$R = \frac{V \cdot (\ln 2) \cdot [P]}{t\,1/2}$$

where R is the rate of release (and also of production in the steady-state); V is the volume of distribution of each NP; [P] represents the plasma concentration determined by radioimmunoassay, and $t\,1/2$ is the half-life of immunoreactive VP in the circulation. The rates of release/production of VP-RNP and OT-RNP estimated in this fashion were: 32 pmol/day/100 g body weight (males) and 41 pmoles/day/100 g body weight (females) for VP-RNP; and 55 pmoles/day/100 g body weight (males) and 81 pmoles/day/100 g body weight (females) for OT-RNP. Rhodes and colleagues [27] used an immunocytochemical approach to determine the num-

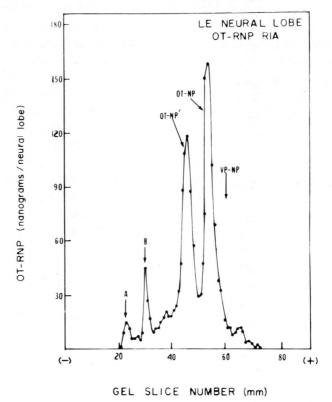

Figure 2. Identification of precursor forms (A, B) in neurosecretory granules from rat neural lobes by RIA for oxytocin-associated rat neurophysin. RIA was performed on eluates from 1-mm strips of a 10% polyacrylamide gel. Electrophoresis was performed at pH 9.5. The positions of oxytocin-associated rat neurophysin (OT-RNP), a metabolite (OT-RNP'), and vasopressin-associated neurophysin (VP-RNP) all located by comassiablue staining, are indicated.

ber of neurons producing NPs, VP, and OT in the rat hypothalamus. Their evaluation gave approximately 4000 for each cell type, and if we assume that about 75 % of these neurons send axons to the neural lobe, then the rate of synthesis of NPs (and VP, OT) per 10^6 cells can be estimated (by coupling the results of our study with theirs) to be about 10 and 15 nmole/day/10^6 cells for VP-RNP, and 20 and 30 nmole/day/10^6 cells for OT-RNP. The molar quantities of each hormone and its corresponding NP stored in the neural lobe are approximately the same, and this appears to be true not only for mature rats, but throughout different stages of postnatal development [4, 28]. A small amount of precursor also appears to be present in the neural lobe, and this has been demonstrated by Russell and co-workers [11] in crude extracts of the gland, and by us for OT-RNP precursor(s) as a component of isolated neurosecretory granules (Figure 2). As the contents of NSG are released by exocytosis of the granules, it is therefore likely that a small amount of the precursors (molecular sizes ~ 20,000 daltons) of vasopressinergic and oxytocinergic neurons are released into the circulation, although this probably represents a very small fraction of the total amounts of hormones and neurophysins released.

Since the neurophysins and hormones are formed in NSG from precursors by proteolysis, then at least one proteolytic enzyme would be expected to be a component of these granules. We, in fact, have demonstrated the presence of an enzyme(s) in an isolated fraction of NSG and found it to be entirely responsible for metabolic products formed from the neurophysins *in situ*. All of these metabolic conversions from purified VP-NPs and OT-NPs by this enzyme at pH 5 have been demonstrated *in vitro* using preparation of isolated NSG [4, 29, 30]. The fact that *in vitro* conversions occur at a pH similar to that measured to be the intragranular pH indicates that the enzyme(s) is active *within NSG*. We found that the enzyme converts OT-RNP to its chief metabolite, OT-RNP', by cleaving a Phe-Ser bond and liberating a small C-terminal peptide, and this has now been confirmed by availability of the amino acid sequence data for OT-RNP and OT-RNP' [31, 32]. On the other hand, it seems to liberate an N-terminal peptide fragment(s) from VP-RNP to form a metabolite VP-RNP'. The similarity of the enzyme(s) to α-chymotrypsin was shown by the ability of α-chymotrypsin at pH 7.6 (a suitable pH for this latter enzyme) to liberate protein and peptide products from purified VP-RNP and OT-RNP which seem to be identical to those products obtained with the enzyme(s) of the granules at pH 4.5. *Unlike* α-chymotrypsin, however, the enzyme(s) of the granules is an acid proteinase and displays maximal activity in the range pH 4.0 to 5.5, and has little to no activity above pH 6.5 and below pH 3.0 [4, 29, 33, 34]. We have further shown that α-chymotrypsin at pH 7.6 is capable of generating all identified NPs of ox and human neural lobe when incubated *in vitro* with purified proteins thought to represent the primary forms of VP-NP and OT-NP in these species. The enzyme(s) of NSG also appears to be present throughout postnatal development in the rat as evidenced by the presence of OT-RNP′ at all stages [4]. The nature of the enzyme(s) of the granules, and its location within NSG make it a possible candidate responsible for the formation of NPs, VP and OT from prohormones. This is now supported by features of the derived amino acid sequence of the precursor of vasopressinergic neurons (Figure 1): if the entire precursor is packaged into NSG, an enzyme similar to the one we have described would be required to cleave the Ala-Cys bond joining hormone to leader peptide. Smyth and Massey [35] have also described fragments of prohormone which would result from Leu-Leu bond cleavages and could arise from the action of the enzyme; and it is also conceivable that our enzyme splits at the Val-Arg bond of the precursor to liberate the NP structure from the C-terminal glycopeptide. Nevertheless, it is clear that enzymes other than the one we have described would also be necessary to produce NPs, VP and OT as final products of the precursor. The requirements are an enzyme to cleave a Gly-Gly bond with amidation of the Gly [9] position of the hormone liberated by such a cleavage [36] and an arylamidase-type activity [37] for fully liberating the NPs; or a trypsin/carboxypeptidase B combination as seen in pancreatic β-cells [38, 39].

The neurosecretory granules of magnocellular neurons are therefore seen to contain precursor, hormone, neurophysin, and other products of proteolysis of the precursor; and more than one proteolytic enzyme responsible for the generation of secretory products from precursor.

3. FACTORS CONTROLLING RELEASE OF NEUROPHYSINS

Neurophysins are released when VP and OT are released. Hence, those factors influencing release of the hormones will also alter circulating levels of neurophysins. The control of VP and OT release from the neurohypophysis has been the subject of extensive reviews [40–42]. The principal physiological control mechanisms for the release of VP (and VP-NP) involve serum osmolality and blood volume changes. An increase in serum osmolality activates osmoreceptors in the hypothalamus stimulating the production/release of the hormone and its neurophysin. This stimulus also causes an increase in production/release of oxytocin and OT-NP [24, 26]. A decrease in blood volume of more than 10% decreases inhibitory impulses to the hypothalamus from atrial receptors and arterial baroreceptors, and this results in a large rise in the production/release from vasopressinergic neurons, but not from oxytocinergic neurons. Nicotine is a stimulus for VP release in animals [8, 9] but not in human subjects who smoke cigarettes regularly [9, 43]. Estrogens are potent stimulants of OT and OT-NP release but have little effect on VP and VP-NP secretion [8, 9]. Release from vasopressinergic neurons also appears to be under the influence of dopamine [44].

4. CLEARANCE OF NEUROPHYSINS

Neurophysins are cleared from the circulation chiefly by the kidneys. In studies conducted on the clearance of rat neurophysins in conscious rats (North and Gellai, unpublished data) we found that very little of this removal (<5%) is by filtration. When ^{125}I-RNPs were injected into rats almost no immunoreactive material was present in urine collected from a bladder catheter – the tracer was in the form of small peptides appearing maximally at times >60 minutes, and some animals sacrificed 20 minutes post-injection showed >85% of the radioactivity located in the kidneys. These data point to cells of the kidneys almost exclusively taking up RNPs from blood, degrading them, and then *secreting* breakdown products into the tubules for removal in the urine.

5. CHARACTERIZATION OF HUMAN NEUROPHYSINS AND DEVELOPMENT OF RIAs [9]

The purification of two human neurophysins was achieved by processing extracts from 5000 human pituitary glands provided by S. Raiti of the National Pituitary Agency. These were characterized as VP-HNP and OT-HNP by their differential association with hormones in human pituitaries and by their specific release in response to different stimuli. They were coupled to bovine thyroglobulin and used to raise antibodies, which in turn were used to develop specific RIAs. Two antisera are effective in assays at dilutions of 1:20,000 and 1:100,000 for VP-HNP and OT-HNP, respectively. The dose range for measurement in the original assays was 5 picograms (0.5 fmole) to 320 picograms (32 fmole) and this made them 1 to 2 orders of magnitude more sensitive than other reported assays for these proteins. Recent modifications in assay procedure have now improved this sensitivity for both assays so that measurements can be performed in the range of 2 picograms (0.2 fmole) to 80 picograms (8 fmole). The cross-reaction of OT-HNP in the assay for VP-HNP is <2%, and the cross-reaction of VP-HNP in the assay for OT-HNP is <5%. Both assays can be used without interference to measure neurophysins in crude tissue extracts and in unextracted plasma and urine.

6. HUMAN NEUROPHYSINS IN PLASMA [9]

The plasma levels of HNPs obtained for 20 healthy subjects (10 males and 10 females) using the above assays were 73 ± 5 pg/ml for VP-HNP and 283 ± 30 pg/ml for OT-HNP. Similar values to these were reported by Pullan and co-workers [43]. The range of values was from < 50 to 132 pg/ml for VP-HNP and from 136 to 562 pg/ml for OT-HNP, and no significant difference was found between sexes. Posture seems to have no influence on HNP levels in plasma.

Since nicotine is reported to be a strong stimulant for the release of vasopressin [45] (and because many patients with SCCL are smokers) we examined the effect of smoking two filtered cigarettes (1.3 mg nicotine/cigarette) in 15 minutes on plasma HNPs in nonsmokers, occasional smokers (< 1 cigarette/week) and habitual smokers. Test samples were taken 10 minutes beforehand, and at 5-minute intervals for 40 minutes after smoking commenced. In nonsmokers and occasional smokers, cigarette smoking was found to cause a 2- to 3-fold increase in plasma values of VP-HNP (but not OT-HNP), and values for this HNP peaked 15–20 minutes after smoking commenced. However, smoking had no significant effect on the levels of VP-HNP or OT-HNP in habitual smokers. In this respect our findings are similar to those reported by Pullan *et al.* [43].

Pathological states which give rise to the syndrome of inappropriate secretion of antidiuretic hormone (SIADH) have been claimed to increase circulating levels of one HNP but not the other [43, 45]. This syndrome is characterized by hyponatremia and high urine osmolality. For 18 patients with SIADH we found that plasma VP-HNP was elevated from 3.3 to 650 times normal. One patient whose SIADH was thought to be due to alcoholism had a VP-HNP value of 456 pg/ml associated with a serum sodium of 103 mEq/liter, and this normalized to 118 pg/ml following treatment when his serum sodium had risen to 134 mEq/liter.

Robinson [45] has shown that estrogen is a strong stimulus for the release of one HNP, but not the other, and this was also our finding [9]. Women taking estrogen-containing oral contraceptives had plasma OT-HNP concentrations at least 4 times the mean value for subjects on no medication (2031 ± 377 pg/ml); but all had normal levels of VP-HNP.

Both HNPs concentrations in plasma are raised in patients with lithium-induced nephrogenic diabetes insipidus [9, 43]. In the one patient examined by us with this condition, the plasma levels were 339 pg/ml for VP-HNP and 3788 pg/ml for OT-HNP. These elevated levels are thought to result from increased release, but it is also possible that impaired kidney function decreases the rates at which HNPs are removed from the circulation (see above).

7. HUMAN NEUROPHYSINS AS POSSIBLE TUMOR MARKERS FOR SMALL CELL
   CARCINOMA OF THE LUNG

Small cell carcinoma of the lung is often associated with the ectopic production of peptide hormones such as ACTH, calcitonin, ADH, and oxytocin [25, 46–48]; and this tumor biosynthesis might proceed by integrated steps similar to those occurring in normal endocrine tissue.

It was on this premise that we set out to examine the incidence of ectopic production of HNPs by small cell carcinoma and to evaluate them as tumor markers [49]. For our evaluation we chose an approach which we have now adopted as a model for this type of investigation. This entails that initial plasma samples are obtained from patients following diagnosis and before they commence therapy. Thereafter, test samples are taken during treatment, *before* each cycle of therapy. Such an approach appears to eliminate the influence that different therapeutic regimens could have on circulating levels of HNPs, and this might also be true for most other tumor markers. An intensive follow-up during treatment seems to us desirable if measurements of the ectopic product are going to be of eventual clinical benefit. The criterion used to identify ectopic production of HNPs in patients before treatment was the presence of elevated plasma levels which were greater than 3 times the mean for normal subjects in the absence of conditions known to increase release from the pituitary or decrease clearance. Such conditions have been reviewed by Robertson [42] and Fenestril [50], and include heart disease, thyroid disease, kidney disease, and adrenal insufficiency. The cut-off values were 220 pg/ml for VP-HNP and 850 pg/ml for OT-HNP (> 4 SDs and > 3 SDs above the normal means for VP-HNP and OT-HNP, respectively). Concentrations of HNPs between 2 and 3 times normal presented us with an intermediate range (> 2 SDs above the normal means for both proteins) and patients with pretherapy values in this range were categorized as having tumors that were possible secretors, although follow-up data indicate that most of these individuals behaved as if they did not have HNP-secreting tumors.

The incidence of ectopic production of HNPs using the above criteria has now been examined for 151 patients. Of these patients, 65% (96) had significantly elevated plasma levels of one, or both, HNPs before therapy (HNP-secreting tumors); 24% (36) had HNP values in the normal range (nonsecreting tumors); and the remaining 13% (19) had values 2-3 times normal (possible HNP-secreting tumors). More specifically, 72 patients (48%) of the 151 had tumors that secreted VP-HNP, and 45 (30%) had tumors that secreted OT-HNP. Of the HNP-secreting tumors 22, (15%) produced both HNPs. The overall incidence of HNP production by small cell tumors was similar for males (62%) and females (66%).

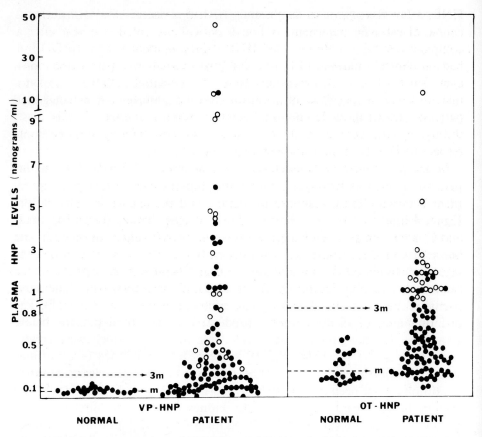

Figure 3. Plasma concentrations of VP-HNP and OT-HNP, determined by RIA, in 20 normal volunteers and 103 patients with small cell carcinoma of the lung at the time of diagnosis. Each person is represented by a single circle for each substance. The mean values of VP-HNP and OT-HNP for healthy volunteers (M) and three times these means (3M) are given, the latter being the lower cut-off which defined the presence of HNP-secreting tumors. O, values for individuals who had both NPs elevated (> 3 times normal). Note the broken scale on the ordinate.

Plasma HNPs have so far been followed in 103 patients who were undergoing a course of combination chemotherapy and radiation therapy. The values of HNPs for these patients before they commenced therapy are illustrated in Figure 3. These patients subsequently had blood samples taken for analysis by RIA just before each therapy session. So far all have been followed through at least two cycles of treatment, while a few have been followed as long as two years. They comprised 67 secretors, 25 nonsecretors, and 11 possible secretors. Patients with nonsecreting tumors maintained normal HNP levels regardless of the clinically assessed course of their disease, with four exceptions. One had a rise in both HNPs following development of massive ascites, one with normal levels for 2 years had a rise in

HNPs a few days prior to death, and one had a rise in OT-HNP during a course of estrogen treatment. A fourth patient presented one year after a complete remission with elevated HNP values, dementia, and SIADH but had no clinical evidence of tumor. No post-mortem was performed, however. Since all of these exceptions have an associated pathology, or have increases due to the effect of a known stimulant, we have concluded that patients classified as having nonsecreting tumors remain in this class throughout the course of their disease – that nonsecreting tumors (with respect to HNPs) remain nonsecreting tumors.

*In sharp contrast to non*secretors *were secretors of HNPs.* For all the patients defined as having HNP-secreting tumors there was a good agreement between clinical response to therapy and the change in HNP levels. Figure 4 illustrates this correlation. Values during therapy (black bars in A and C) are given as a percentage of pretherapy HNP values (open bars); the black bars in B represent values during early recurrent disease as a percentage of those found during remission (shaded bars). For all patients so far examined with high plasma levels of VP-HNP (secretors) who underwent partial remission (defined as a >50% reduction in the sum of the products of 2 diameters of all measurable lesions) or complete remission (no meas-

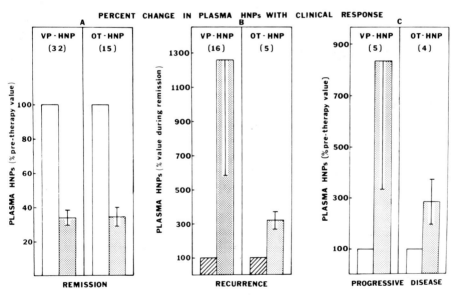

Figure 4. Changes in plasma HNPs during therapy for patients having small cell carcinoma and elevated HNP(s) before treatment. The mean values ($\pm$1 SEM) for the number of patients indicated in parentheses are expressed either as a percentage of pretherapy values (A and C) or as a percentage of values during remission (B). (A) patients who underwent partial or complete remission; (B) patients who had recurrent disease after a previous remission; (C) patients who had no objective response to therapy and showed evidence of progressive disease.

urable lesions or clinically evident para-endocrine disorder), there was a coincident 2- to 20-fold reduction (1 log) of plasma VP-HNP. Elevated plasma levels of OT-HNP were affected in the same manner as VP-HNP levels (2- to 30-fold reductions). For patients with both HNPs in the range for secretors before therapy, clinical remission was associated with reductions in the levels of both proteins. In cases where only one HNP was elevated > 3 times before therapy, it was only this HNP that underwent significant change during remission. For all patients with elevated HNP(s) (> 3 times) who had progressive disease without objective remission, progressive disease was accompanied by increases in HNPs, but only the HNP(s) that was elevated before treatment. Some patients did not experience either a remission or disease progression during the first three cycles of therapy, and their condition during this time was regarded as stable. None of these patients who had HNP-secreting tumors experienced a large rise or fall in their HNP values. However, several showed significant increases or decreases (1.4 to 1.8 times) which could indicate that the RIAs, because of their sensitivity, can register changes in tumor volume too small to be detected by clinical assessment.

The influence of tumor recurrence on plasma HNPs has been assessed in patients with HNP-secreting tumors who had undergone partial or complete remission. In all cases, recurrent disease was associated with increases over remission values in the HNP(s) that was elevated before therapy. Moreover, a significant rise above remission values (> 1.4 times) always preceded clinical recognition of recurrent disease by 3–12 weeks. The one apparent exception to HNP levels always predicting recurrent disease was a patient with 4 times normal VP-HNP before therapy who had a 2-fold reduction in this value coincident with a complete clinical remission. The patient has now been followed for more than 2 years with test samples taken monthly. Although he still shows no signs of a relapse, VP-HNP levels rose to 7 times normal five months after commencing treatment and have remained elevated (> 3 times normal) since that time. OT-HNP levels in this patient were initially normal, but these rose concomitantly with VP-HNP values to 6 times normal and have also remained high (> 3 times normal). The latter finding suggests that a nontumor-related condition could be responsible but such a condition is not yet clearly evident. However, the general pattern observed for patients with high pretherapy levels of VP-HNP is shown in Figure 5. One patient (Figure 5A) had an initial plasma VP-HNP which was 50 times normal and this fell coincident with a complete remission to a value about 6 times normal. During remission plasma levels started to climb and when they had reached 24 times normal the patient was assessed as still in complete clinical remission, except for a possible rib abnormality seen on a bone scan. Recurrent disease was clearly demonstrated after

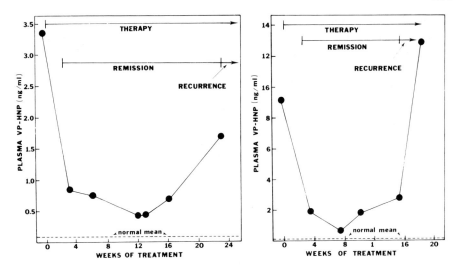

Figure 5. Change in plasma VP-HNP for two patients during treatments for small cell carcinoma, demonstrating the fall in elevated levels characteristic of clinically assessed remission (in both cases, complete remission) and the rise above remission values which typically preceded clinical recognition of recurrent disease. - - - -, mean plasma VP-HNP concentration found for 20 healthy individuals.

another 3 weeks. OT-HNP levels remained normal in this patient throughout treatment. The other patient (Figure 5B) had initial plasma VP-HNP which was 125 times normal and this also fell with complete remission to 9 times normal. VP-HNP then started to rise, first to 25 times normal, and then to 38 times normal when he redeveloped SIADH concurrent with diagnosis of recurrent disease: VP-HNP then rose to 176 times normal. For this patient OT-HNP was elevated at 4 times normal before treatment, fell to 1.5 times normal during remission, and finally rose to 5 times normal.

With reference to RIAs for HNP being able to detect residual tumor above, about half of the patients defined as having HNP-secreting tumors have initial values of one or both HNPs less than 5 times normal, and during partial or complete remission these values fall into the normal range. In such cases we would anticipate that it may still be possible to distinguish ectopic production from normal production by applying qualitative rather than quantitative analysis (see below), or by developing provocative or inhibiting tests (e.g., water restriction or water-loading) [51].

One valuable advantage of monitoring HNPs is the possible use for short-term appraisal of new regimens used in treatment. This was exemplified by one patient who was initially given treatment which involved combination chemotherapy before prophylactic brain radiation therapy. This patient experienced a fall in elevated VP-HNP with remission following chemotherapy, but levels rose significantly during radiation treatments to his brain. When chemotherapy was reinstated, the values again decreased. Subsequent patients were given simultaneous chemotherapy and radiation therapy.

The potential uses of data on plasma HNPs for monitoring the effectiveness of treatment in patients with small cell carcinoma of the lung has led us to seek answers to the following questions: (1) Is there a relationship between initially elevated HNP(s) and the staging of small cell carcinoma into limited and extensive disease?; (2) Is there a relationship between production of HNP(s) and tumor cell subtype?; (3) Is ectopic production of HNP(s) unique to small cell carcinoma of the lung?; and (4) Do changes in plasma HNP(s) provide a true guide to changes in tumor burden?

8. ECTOPIC PRODUCTION OF HNP(s) BY SMALL CELL TUMORS AND STAGING

We have reviewed data on 103 patients to compare secretory status and the staging of the disease and this analysis is given in Table 1. Definition of the stage was according to Cancer and Acute Leukemia, Study Group B, criteria: patients with limited disease had detectable tumor confined to the lung, mediastinum and ipselateral or contralateral supraclavicular lymph nodes; while patients with extensive disease had tumor that extended beyond these confines. Evaluation for sites of metastatic disease employed technetium liver and bone scans, technetium brain scans or computerized axial tomography, analysis of bone marrow aspirates and biopsies, and chest X-ray.

Of patients with extensive disease, 82% had one, or both HNPs in the secretor range (>3 times normal) before therapy, and this compared with 41% of patients with limited disease. The lower incidence for limited disease could be due to a smaller tumor burden in these patients, or to the HNPs being molecular markers of a tumor subtype which shows a greater ability to metastasize. However, of these two possibilities, the first seems

Table 1. Pretherapy HNP secretory status and staging.

Elevated plasma HNP (>3 times normal)	Percentage incidence	
	Limited disease	Extensive disease
VP-HNP elevated only	24%	39%
OT-HNP elevated only	10%	15%
Both HNP elevated	7%	28%
Total patients	42	61

Table 2. Pretherapy HNP secretory status and prognosis.

HNP secretory status	Limited disease			Extensive disease		
	Remission		Median survival	Remission		Median survival
	% complete	% partial	(months)	% complete	% partial	(months)
Secretors	65	24	9.3	8	28	6.1
Nonsecretors	63	13	9.5	11	33	6.5
Possible secretors	22	78	10.0	50	0	5.8

unlikely because results from serial measurements where tumor burden increased with time support the view 'once a nonsecretor always a nonsecretor'. As the prognosis for extensive disease is poorer than for limited disease [52, 53], then indirect support for the second of the above possibilities might be gained if patients with HNP-secreting tumors within each staging group were found to have a poorer prognosis than patients with non-HNP-secreting tumors. However, examination of data for 103 patients showed that there was no clear prognostic difference between secreting and nonsecreting tumors, either in terms of the percentage of patients exhibiting a positive response or in median survival (Table 2).

9. HNP SECRETORY STATUS AND CELL SUBTYPES OF SMALL CELL CARCINOMA OF THE LUNG

In a further analysis of the data gathered on the above 103 patients, we compared the pretherapy elevation (> 3 times normal) with subclassification

Table 3. Pretherapy HNP secretory status and cell subtype.

Staging and secretory status	Cell subtype		
	Lymphocytic	Intermediate	SCCL NOS[a]
Limited disease	18	19	5
Extensive disease	24	26	11
Secretes VP-HNP *alone*	14 (33%)	16 (36%)	4 (25%)
Secretors OT-HNP *alone*	3 (7%)	9 (20%)	1 (6%)
Secretors *both* HNPs	11 (26%)	8 (18%)	1 (6%)
Nonsecretors	8 (19%)	7 (16%)	6 (38%)
Possible secretors	6 (14%)	5 (11%)	4 (25%)

[a] Small cell carcinoma not otherwise specified.

of tumors into lymphocytic cell type, intermediate cell type, and small cell not-otherwise-specified (SCCL NOS) according to the 1979 WHO recommendations. This analysis is shown in Table 3. Although numbers are small, there was no significant difference in secretory status between lymphocytic and intermediate cell subtypes and for these two groups the incidence of HNP secretion was 44% for limited disease and 88% for extensive disease. The incidence of secretion in tumors with unspecified cell subtyping was much lower than this.

10. ECTOPIC PRODUCTION OF VP AND OT BY SMALL CELL CARCINOMA

We developed a dependable method for extracting VP from plasma [54] and found this also suitable for isolating OT for RIA. The method provides a >80% recovery of the peptides from 1.0 ml of plasma. Using RIAs [25, 55] data on plasma levels of *extractable* hormones (i.e., as peptide products, not as larger molecular forms) has been obtained for 18 patients who have also been assessed for ectopic production of HNPs. Prior to treatment, 3 of the patients studied displayed SIADH and had elevated VP-HNP, 4 had elevated VP-HNP, 3 had elevated OT-HNP, 1 had both HNPs elevated, and 10 had normal plasma levels of HNPs. For 9 of 10 patients with normal HNPs (nonsecretors), the corresponding hormone levels were in the normal range (2–4 pg/ml for VP, 2–6 pg/ml for OT). The remaining one of these 8 patients had a normal VP value, but 18 times the normal plasma value of 3.0 pg/ml for OT. For the other patients, in all instances where one or both HNPs were elevated (>3 times normal), the corresponding hormone was also elevated (>3 times normal). However, one patient with elevated VP-HNP and normal OT-HNP had an OT value which was >300 times normal. During treatment the direction of change in hormone levels was generally the same as that of the HNP. Hence, the data while still preliminary suggest that: (1) all tumors secreting VP-HNP and OT-HNP also secrete VP and OT and, therefore, their production by these cells arises from genetic derepression; and (2) the incidence of OT secretion by tumors may be higher than that suggested by the RIA used for OT-HNP. For plasma VP, SIADH was associated with levels of the hormone >14 pg/ml and was no longer apparent when values dropped to <10 pg/ml.

Since each HNP and its hormone are likely generated from a common precursor, and stored and released in molar equivalents by hypothalamic neurons (see Introduction) we expect that plasma levels resulting from normal production should reflect such processing with differences being due to their respective clearances and volumes of distribution. In this respect, we have determined that the plasma molar ratios of VP-HNP and VP in healthy volunteers is between 3 and 6 (North, unpublished data). Our evaluation of the plasma ratios of VP-HNP to VP in three patients with HNP-secreting tumors before and during treatment (Table 4) has shown that this index is outside the normal range, even when plasma concentrations of the secreted material returned to normal following remission in one of the patients. For Patient 1 of Table 4 the NP:hormone ratio was lower than normal before therapy and remained low during remission. At the time of recurrent disease in this patient, and in Patients 2 and 3 who had progressive disease the ratio was abnormally high. In fact, it increased with time in Patient 1. A relatively low value for extractable VP compared to VP-HNP suggests to us that these substances are being secreted principally as a large molecular form(s) – as precursor. Our present knowledge of the production of VP and VP-NP by neurons leads us to believe that such changes may be due to alterations in the levels of intragranular proteolytic enzymes produced by the tumor cells, enzymes normally responsible for the generation of hormones and neurophysins from precursors. Such alterations could be significant if they accompanied increased resistance of tumors to treatment. Further support for qualitative differences between the secretions from tumors and from the hypothalamic neurons has also come from our studies performed on the gel filtration behavior of immunoassayable HNPs. For plasma from healthy individuals we found that almost all of the activity in the assays for HNPs was eluted from columns of Sephadex G-75 in volumes similar to those in which pituitary neurophysins were eluted. Such peaks of activity indicated a molecular size of 15,000 to 20,000 at pH 7.0 and this is consistent with the known tendency of the 10,000 dalton species to form dimers under these conditions (for review see NY Acad Sci, volume 248, 1975). However, in the plasma samples from some tumor patients, a much larger species of HNP(s) was also found. One profile obtained from the plasma of a patient undergoing a relapse and displaying 'big neurophysin' is shown in Figure 6. Yamaji et al. [56] have also demonstrated large glycosylated forms of one HNP in small cell tumors. Both observations suggest that tumors not uncommonly secrete precursor forms of the HNPs as has been shown for the ectopic production of other hormones and hormone-associated substances [46, 48].

11. TUMOR CONTENT OF HNPs

We have examined three tumors classified as nonsecreting and were unable to detect HNP(s) by RIA in acid extracts. However, the extracts from a primary lung tumor and liver metastasis of a secretor of VP-HNP were found to have 8.7 ng/mg acid-soluble protein (0.8 pmole/mg acid-soluble

Table 4. Plasma molar ratios of VP-HNP and VP for three patients with SCCL.

Patient 1					Patient 2					Patient 3				
Time[c] (weeks)	VP-HNP (pg/ml)	VP (pg/ml)	Ratio[a]	C.A.[b]	Time (weeks)	VP-HNP (pg/ml)	VP (pg/ml)	Ratio	C.A.	Time (weeks)	VP-HNP (pg/ml)	VP (pg/ml)	Ratio	C.A.
0	274	30.2	0.9		0	1195	13.3	9.0		0	5925	14.7	40	
9	54	2.8	1.9		1	1067	9.4	11.4		7	10084	83.0	12	PD
12	74	2.9	2.6	CR	8	864	5.2	16.6	S	12	13530	56.4	24	
15	42	27.1	0.2		15	2769	21.2	13.1	PD					
19	155	3.7	4.2		21	6900	36.7	18.8						
23	61	4.5	1.4											
27	244	9.0	2.7											
30	441	8.5	5.2											
39	1862	15.5	12											
44	2576	7.5	34											
47	6088	14	44	RP										
52	6079	17.1	36											
55	12390	29.1	43											
57	15834	29.9	54											

[a] Molar ratio, VP = 1000; VP-HNP = 10,000.
[b] Clinical assessment, CR = complete response, PR = partial response, S = stable, RP = relapse, PD = progressive disease.
[c] Time from initial supply taken one day before starting treatment.

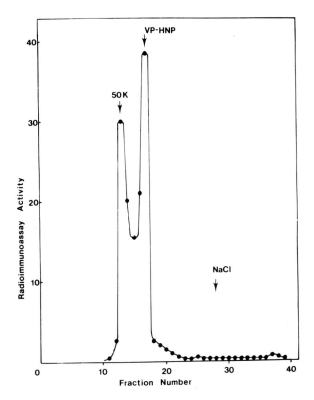

Figure 6. Profile of plasma immunoreactive neurophysins eluted from a column of Sephadex G-75. The plasma sample was from a patient undergoing relapse who had a small cell tumor that produced VP-HNP. The elution volumes for pituitary VP-HNP, NaCl, and a 50,000 dalton protein are indicated. The 50K point was derived from data obtained on standard mixtures of proteins used as molecular weight markers.

protein) and 6.5 ng/mg acid-soluble protein of VP-HNP, and no detectable OT-HNP. A cell line (DMS-217) was developed from a pericardial metastasis taken from the same patient and this cell line after being maintained in culture for two years was found to contain 5.8 ng/mg acid-soluble protein of VP-HNP. These data indicate the presence of low and consistent storage level of secretory product in primary and metastatic disease, and in cell lines derived from such tumors. In fact, for 14 cell lines developed from small cell tumors by Pettengill and Sorenson [57] we have found substantial amounts of OT-HNP, VP-HNP, or both HNPs [57]. It is not yet known how such measurements in media relate to storage or production by these cell lines because a number of variables were not taken into account: cell viability, the stability of the secretory products to possible breakdown by enzymes in the media or secreted by the tumors, and possible feed-back regulation of secretory products on tumor cell activity.

Although the rate of production/release of HNPs by small cell tumor has yet to be measured, we have some indications of what this production/release could be from the studies of George *et al.* [58] and Klein *et al.* [59] who measured production of vasopressin by small cell carcinoma cells. Klein and co-workers estimated the rate of vasopressin production/release to be 1.0 pmoles/hr/mg wet weight of tissue by a monolayer culture, and George and his colleagues obtained a value of 0.17 pmoles/hr/mg wet weight of tissue by slices of tumor tissue *in vitro*. If HNP(s) are produced/released at a similar rate to the hormone(s) (see above) we might expect from these data that amounts of HNP(s) somewhere in the range of 0.2 to 1.0 pmoles are produced each hour by one milligram of tumor cells.

A production of vasopressin (or VP-HNP) of 1.0 pmole/hr/mg tumor cells as found by Klein *et al.* suggests that tumor production of such secretory products is at least two orders of magnitude less than their production by hypothalamic neurons if 10^6 tumor cells are taken weigh about one milligram. It is also of interest to speculate that if the half-lives and volumes of distribution of HNPs in man are similar to those found by us for RNPs in

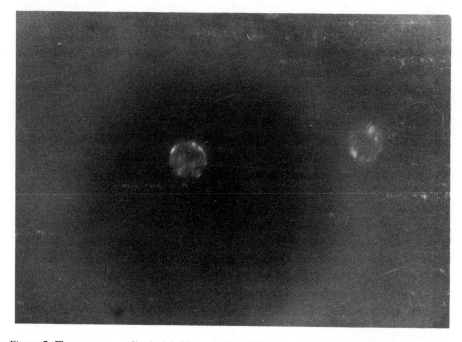

Figure 7. Fluorescence-antibody labelling of DMS 240 cells derived in culture from small cell carcinoma cells. The tissue source was liver, and the patient was earlier described by our assays to have tumor which secreted both HNPs. Cells were found reacted with anti-HNP IgG, and then with fluoroscein-labelled goat-anti-rabbit IgG.

rats, then a 2.0-gm tumor in a 70-kg individual would raise the plasma level of each HNP by approximately 200 pg/ml.

We have performed initial studies designed to localize neurophysins on tumor cells *in vitro* using the fluorescent-antibody technique. In these studies we incubated viable cells of a cell line, DMS-240, with IgG from anti-(OT-HNP) serum, washed the cells in phosphate-buffered saline, and then exposed them to fluorescein-bound goat anti-rabbit IgG. After further washings the cells were visualized under UV-light and showed bright clumps of fluorescence over their surfaces as shown in Figure 7. This was not seen when normal rabbit IgG was used as control. Hence, we now know that antibodies to the HNPs can bind to HNP-secreting cells.

While we have no assurance that tumor production of hormones involves their packaging into subcellular granules, a number of small cell tumors have been described which contain such granules [48]. George and co-workers [58] found electron-dense secretory granules ranging in size from 130 to 240 nm in a small cell tumor which produced vasopressin (ADH). This

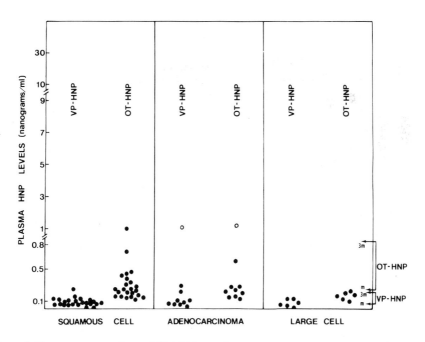

Figure 8. Plasma concentrations of VP-HNP and OT-HNP, determined by RIA, for 39 patients with lung cancer other than small cell carcinoma of the lung at the time of diagnosis. Each person is represented by a single circle for each substance. O, values for individuals with both NPs elevated (> 3 times normal). The mean values of VP-HNP and OT-HNP (M) for healthy individuals and three times these means (3M) are indicated. Note the broken scale on the ordinate.

would support the view that at least some tumors have the capability of processing vasopressin, oxytocin, and neurophysins in the same manner as hypothalamic neurons.

12. PRODUCTION OF HNPs BY TUMORS OTHER THAN SMALL CELL CARCINOMA

We have examined the incidence of elevated plasma HNP(s) for 39 patients with a histological diagnosis of lung cancer other than small cell carcinoma of the lung. Plasma samples from these patients were drawn before therapy was instituted. The biopsy specimens were reviewed by the CALGB reference pathologist for lung cancer who was not aware of the values we obtained in our RIAs. Results for lung cancers are shown in Figure 8. For squamous cell carcinoma, 2 of 23 patients (9%) had elevated values (>3 times normal). One patient had elevated VP-HNP (252 pg/ml; 3.6 times normal), and the other elevated OT-HNP (1020 pg/ml, 4 times normal).

For adenocarcinoma, 3 of 10 patients (30%) had elevated HNP(s). One patient had plasma levels of both neurophysins elevated (VP-HNP, 1098 pg/ml, 15 times normal; OT-HNP, 1261 pg/ml, 5 times normal). This patient had a pericardial tamponade and a serum sodium of 132 milliequivalents/liter, and this may in part explain the elevations. Two other patients had only VP-HNP raised (220 pg/ml, 3 times normal; 298 pg/ml, 4 times normal).

None of the 6 patients with large cell carcinoma had elevated HNP(s) before therapy, and this brought the overall incidence of elevated HNP(s) in lung cancer other than small cell carcinoma to 5 of 39 patients or 13%. These data suggest that a diagnosis of the presence of small cell carcinoma based on the presence of significantly elevated HNP(s) (>3 times normal) in a patient with lung cancer prior to therapy would have an 83% likelihood of being a correct one. This statistical likelihood for a correct diagnosis of the presence of small cell carcinoma is increased to 95% if the cut-off points for ectopically elevated plasma HNPs are made at 300 pg/ml for VP-HNP (4.1 times normal) and 1100 pg/ml for OT-HNP (4.3 times normal).

13. CONCLUSIONS

The study of plasma HNPs in patients with small cell carcinoma of the lung has provided information that there is a probable high incidence of production of these proteins by this tumor type. Since the high incidence seems confined to small cell carcinoma, at least for lung cancers, the presence of highly elevated plasma HNP(s) in a patient should aid diagnosis. Neurophysins seem to be effective monitors of response to therapy for patients with small cell carcinoma, and the RIAs for these substances may therefore afford us a sensitive and reliable method to assess changes in tumor burden that occur during response, enable small amounts of residual tumor to be detected, and to forecast recurrent disease. This in turn, could afford a better evaluation of response to therapy, allowing its description in terms of the changes in tumor marker concentration rather than by current definitions of partial or complete remission, and progressive disease. In this respect we see real potential value in the treatment of extensive disease which has a poor prognosis and where the markers can provide short-term feed-back on the effectiveness of newly introduced regimens. In limited disease, which has a better prognosis, there is also a need for chemical markers to clearly distinguish cases of complete remission and to provide a periodic check on the disease status for such patients. In fact it is conceivable that the recognition of good chemical markers will ultimately result in a redefinition of the biology of the small cell carcinoma evaluated on the basis of the presence or absence of such molecular fingerprints. Evidence for a possible redefinition is seen in the higher incidence of these markers in extensive *versus* limited disease. Here may be a different cell type more likely to be secretory involved in overt metastatic disease at diagnosis. The immediate future offers us an opportunity to localize small cell tumors from whole-body radioscans following injection of ^{131}I-labelled anti-HNPs [59], to target therapy using anti-HNPs and deliver a high pulse of radiation or chemotherapeutic agent directly onto the tumor cells [60–62], and to use fluorescence-labelled anti-HNPs to identify tumor cells in pleural fluid and CSF biopsies.

We believe that the long-term benefit derived from studying markers such as the HNPs will be an enhanced understanding of tumor biosynthesis and of the process of carcinogenesis. In common with normal production by hypothalamic neurons, tumor production shows (1) neurophysins are synthesized via larger molecular forms, or precursors, which they likely share with oxytocin or vasopressin; (2) the precursor of VP-HNP and VP is at least in certain cases, glycosylated; (3) the ectopic products may be released from subcellular granules by exocytosis; and (4) the battery of enzymes necessary to generate neurophysins and hormones from precursors must be co-produced with the precursors because the hormone(s) are often biologically active. However, small cell tumor production appears to differ from production by neurons because, (1) the rates of synthesis/release by tumors seem to be about two orders of magnitude less than by neurons; (2) there appears to be a much smaller storage of products in tumors compared to neurons (which may reflect a smaller rate of synthesis); (3) several tumors show the capacity to produce both hormones (although this may be due to cell heterogeneity in tumors); (4) tumor production seems to be chiefly autonomous; and (5) the conversion of precursors to hormones and neurophysins within tumor cells is not tightly regulated because larger forms are often released, and because the ratio of immunologically intact VP and VP-HNP resulting from production by tumors can show large changes with time.

Neurophysins, therefore, may provide us with many ways of effectively managing small cell carcinoma of the lung. However, a determination of their true value in this regard must await the outcome of a large body of work still to be accomplished.

ACKNOWLEDGMENTS

This work was supported in part by US Public Health Service Research Grants CA 19613, Am 08469, and Contract N01-CN-55199 from the National Cancer Institute. William G. North is the recipient of USPHS Research Career Development Award CA-00552.

We wish to thank Gail Hardy, Susan Kullmann, Teresa Mitchell and Gary Allen for providing excellent technical assistance.

REFERENCES

1. Sachs H, Fawcett P, Takabatake Y, Portanova R: Biosynthesis and release of vasopressin and neurophysin. Rec Prog Horm Res 25:447–491, 1969.
2. Pickering BT, Jones CW, Burford GD, McPherson M, Swann RR, Heap PF, Morris JF: The role of neurophysin proteins: suggestions from the study of their transport and turnover. Ann NY Acad Sci 248:15–35, 1975.
3. Gainer H, Sarne Y, Brownstein MJ: Biosynthesis and axonal transport of rat neurohypophysial proteins and peptides. J Cell Biol 73: 366–381, 1977.
4. North WG, LaRochelle FT Jr, Morris JF, Sokol HW, Valtin H: Biosynthetic specificity of neurons producing neurohypophysial principles. In: Current Studies of Hypothalamic Function. Lederis K, Veale WH (eds)., Basel: Karger, 1978, pp 62–76.
5. Russell JT, Brownstein MJ, Gainer H: Trypsin liberates an arginine vasopressin-like peptide and neurophysin from a M_r 20,000 putative common precursor. Proc Natl Acad Sci 76:6086–6090, 1979.
6. Pickering BT, North WG: Biochemical and functional aspects of magnocellular neurons and hypothalamic diabetes insipidus. Ann NY Acad Sci, 1982 (in press).
7. Land H, Schutz G, Schmale H, Richter D: Nucleotide sequence of cloned DNA encoding bovine arginine vasopressin-neurophysin II precursor. Nature 295:299–303, 1982.
8. Robinson AG, Haluszczak C, Wilkins JA, Heullmantel AB, Watson CG: Physiological control of two neurophysins in humans. J Clin Endocrinol Metab 44:330, 1977.

9. North WG, LaRochelle FT Jr, Melton J, Mills RC: Isolation and partial characterization of two human neurophysins: Their use in the development of specific radioimmunoassays. J Clin Endocrinol Metab 51: 884–891, 1980.

10. Valtin H, Sokol HW (eds): NY Acad Sci 'The Brattleboro Rat', 1982, vol. 394.

11. Russell JT, Brownstein MJ, Gainer H: Time course of appearance and release of [^{35}S]cysteine labelled neurophysins and peptides in the neurohypophysis. Brain Research 205:299–311, 1981.

12. Schmale H, Leipold B, Richter D: Cell-free translation of bovine hypothalamic mRNA. FEBS Letters 108:311–316, 1979.

13. Schmale H, Richter D: Immunological identification of a common precursor to arginine vasopressin and neurophysin II synthesized by in vitro translation of bovine hypothalamic mRNA. Proc Natl Acad Sci 78:766–769, 1981.

14. Guidice LC, Chaiken IM: Immunological and chemical identification of a neurophysin-containing protein coded by messenger RNA from bovine hypothalamus. Proc Natl Acad Sci 76:3800–3804, 1979.

15. Lin C, Joseph-Bravo P, Sherman T, McKelvy J: Cell-free synthesis of putative neurophysin precursors from rat and mouse hypothalamic poly (A)-RNA. Biochem Biophys Res Commun 89:943–950, 1979.

16. Russell JT, Brownstein MJ, Gainer H: Biosynthesis of vasopressin, oxytocin and neurophysins: Isolation and characterization of two common precursors (propressophysin and prooxyphysin). Endocrinology 107:1880–1891, 1980.

17. Tasso F, Rua S, Picard D: Cytochemical duality of neurosecretory material in the hypothalamo-posthypophysial system of the rat as related to hormone content. Cell Tiss Res 180:11–29, 1977.

18. Rosenoir JC, North WG, Moore GJ: Putative precursors of vasopressin, oxytocin, and neurophysins in the rat hypothalamus. Endocrinology 109:1067–1072, 1981.

19. Lauber M, Camier M, Cohen P: Immunological and biochemical characterization of distinct high molecular weight forms of neurophysin and somatostatin in mouse hypothalamic extracts. FEBS Letters 97:343–347, 1979.

20. Nicolas P, Camier M, Lauber M, Masse MJO, Mohring J, Cohen P: Immunological identification of high molecular weight forms common to bovine neurophysin and vasopressin. Proc Natl Acad Sci 77:2587–2591, 1980.

21. Cannata, MA, Morris JF: Changes in the appearance of hypothalamo-neurohypophysial neurosecretory granules associated with their maturation. J Endocr 57:531–538, 1973.

22. Russell JT, Holtz RW: Measurement of pH and membrane potential in isolated neurosecretory vesicles from bovine neurohypophyses. J Biol Chem 256:5950–5953, 1981.

23. Morris JF: Hormone storage in individual neurosecretory granules of the pituitary gland: a quantitative ultrastructural approach to hormone storage in the neural lobe. J Endocr 68:209–224, 1976.

24. North WG, LaRochelle FJ Jr, Hardy GR: Development of radioimmunoassays to individual rat neurophysins. J Endocrinol (in press), 1982.

25. Dreifuss JJ: A review of neurosecretory granules: their contents and mechanism of release. NY Acad Sci 248:184–201, 1975.

26. North WG, Gellai M, Hardy G: Oxytocin and oxytocin-associated neurophysin evaluation by RIA in the Brattleboro rat. Ann NY Acad Sci 394:167–172, 1982.

27. Rhodes CH, Morrell JI, Pfaff DW: Immunohistochemical analysis of magnocellular elements in rat hypothalamus: Distribution and number of cells containing neurophysin, oxytocin and vasopressin. J Comp Neurol 198:45–64, 1981.

28. Valtin, H, North WG, LaRochelle FT Jr, Sokol HW, Morris JF: Biochemical and anatomical aspects of ADH production. In: Proc VII Int Cong Nephrol. Bergeron M (ed). Basel: Karger, 1978, pp 313–320.

168

29. North WG, Valtin H: The purification of rat neurophysins by a method of preparative polyacrylamide gel electrophoresis. Analyt Biochem 78:436–450, 1976.
30. North WG, Valtin H, Morris JF, LaRochelle FT Jr: Evidence for metabolic conversions of rat neurophysins within neurosecretory granules of the hypothalamo-neurohypophysial system. Endocrinology 101:110–118, 1977.
31. North WG, Mitchell TI: Evolution of neurophysin proteins: The partial sequence of rat neurophysins. FEBS Letters 126:41–44, 1981.
32. Chauvet M-T, Chauvet J, Acher R: Identification of rat neurophysins: Complete amino acid sequences of MSEL- and VLDV-neurophysins. Biochem Biophys Res Commun 103:595–603, 1981.
33. North WG, Valtin H, Morris JF: Evidence for enzymatic (metabolic) conversion of rat neurophysins. Clin Res 24: 429A, 1976.
34. North WG, Morris JF, LaRochelle FT Jr, Valtin H: Enzymatic interconversions of neurophysins. In: Neurophypophysis. Moses AM, Share L (eds). Basel: Karger, 1977, pp 43–52.
35. Smyth DG, Massey D: A new glycopeptide in pig, ox and sheep pituitary. Biochem Biophys Res Commun 87:1006–1010, 1979.
36. Pickering BR: The molecules of neurosecretion: their formation, transport and release. Prog Horm Res 45:161–179, 1976.
37. Marks N, Lajtha A: Protein and polypeptide breakdown. In: Handbook of Neurochemistry 5A. Lajtha A (ed). New York: Plenum, 1971, p 49.
38. Steiner DF: Peptide hormone precursors: biosynthesis, processing and significance. In: Peptide Hormones. Parsons JA (ed). London: MacMillan, 1976, pp 49–64.
39. Fletcher DJ, Quigley J, Baver EJ, Noe BD: Characterization of pro-insulin and proglucagon-converting activities in isolated islet secretory granules. J Cell Biol 90: 312–322, 1981.
40. Sawyer WH, Knobil E (eds): Handbook of Physiology, volume IV, The Pituitary Gland and its neuroendocrine control, Part I. American Physiological Society, 1974.
41. Moses AM, Miller M (eds): Neurohypophysis. Basel: Karger, 1977.
42. Robertson GL: The regulation of vasopressin function in health and disease. Rec Prog Horm Res 33: 333–385, 1977.
43. Pullan PT, Clappison BH, Johnston CI: Plasma vasopressin and human neurophysins in physiological and pathological states associated with changes in vasopressin secretion. J Clin Endocrinol Metab 49:580–587, 1979.
44. Forsling ML, Iverson LL, Lightman SL: Dopamine and enkephalin directly inhibit vasopressin release from the neurohypophysis. J Physiol 319:66P, 1981.
45. Robinson AG: Neurophysins and their physiological significance. In: Neuroendocrinology, Krieger DT, Hughes JC (eds)., Sunderland: Sinauer Assoc Inc, 1980, p 149.
46. Yalow RS: Big ACTH and bronchogenic carcinoma. Ann Rev Med 30:241–248, 1979.
47. Wallach SR, Royston T, Taetle R, Wohl H, Deftos LJ: Plasma calcitonin as a marker of disease activity in patients with small cell carcinoma of the lung. J Clin Endocrinol Metab 53:602–606, 1981.
48. Rees LH: The biosynthesis of hormones by non-endocrine tumors – a review. J Endocr 67:143–174, 1975.
49. North WG, Maurer LH, Valtin H, O'Donnell J: Human neurophysins as potential tumor markers for small cell carcinoma of the lung: Application of specific radioimmunoassays for vasopressin-associated and oxytocin-associated neurophysins. J Clin Endocrinol Metab 51:892–896, 1980.
50. Fenestril DD: Hyposmolar syndromes. In: Disturbances in the Body Fluid Osmolality. Andreoli TE, Grantham JJ, Rector FC Jr (eds). Bethesda: American Physiological Society, 1977, p 267.

51. Miller M, Moses AM: Radioimmunoassay of urinary antidiuretic hormone in man: Response to water load and dehydration in normal subjects. J Clin Endocrinol Metab 34:537–545, 1972.
52. Maurer LH, Tulloh M, Weiss RB, Blom J, Leone L, Glidewell O, Pajak TF: A randomized combined modality trial in small cell carcinoma of the lung. Cancer 45:30–39, 1980.
53. Greco FA, Richardson RL, Snell JD, Stroup SL, Oldham RK: Small cell cancer: Complete remission and improved survival. Am J Med 66:625–630, 1979.
54. LaRochelle FT Jr, North WG, Stern P: A new extraction of arginine vasopressin from blood: the use of octadecasilyl-silica. Pflugers Arch Eur J Physiol 387:79–81, 1980.
55. North WG, LaRochelle FT Jr, Haldar J, Sawyer WH, Valtin H: Characterization of an antiserum used in a radioimmunoassay for arginine-vasopressin: implications for reference standards. Endocrinology 103: 1976–1984, 1978.
56. Yamaji T, Ishibashi M, Katayama S: Nature of the immunoreactive neurophysins in ectopic vasopressin-producing oat-cell carcinomas of the lung. J Clin Invest 68:388–398, 1981.
57. Pettengill OS, Sorenson GD: Tissue culture and in vitro characteristics in small cell carcinoma. In: Small Cell Lung Cancer, Greco FA, Oldham RK, Bunn PA Jr (eds). New York: Grune and Stratton, 1981.
58. George JM, Capen CC, Philips AS: Biosynthesis of vasopressin in vitro and ultrastructure of a bronchogenic carcinoma. Patient with syndrome of inappropriate secretion of antidiuretic hormone. J Clin Invest 51:141–148, 1972.
59. Klein LA, Rabson AS, Worksman J: In vitro synthesis of vasopressin by lung tumor cells. Surg Forum 20:231–233, 1969.
60. Goldenberg DM, DeLand F, Kim E, Bennett S, Primus FJ, Van Nagell JR, Estes N, DeSimone P, Rayburn P: Use of radiolabelled antibodies to carcinoembryonic antigen for the detection and localization of diverse cancers by external photoscanning. New Eng J Med 298:1384–1388, 1978.
61. Goldenberg DM, Kim EE, DeLand FH, Bennett S, Primus J: Radioimmunodetection of cancer with radioactive antibodies to carcinoembryonic antigen. Cancer Research 40:2984–2992, 1980.
62. Glennie MJ, Stevenson GT: Univalent antibodies kill tumor cells in vitro and in vivo. Nature 295:712-714, 1982.

10. The Potential Role of Surgery in the Contemporary Combined Modality Management of Small Cell Anaplastic Lung Cancer

ROBERT L. COMIS

1. INTRODUCTION

Prior to the development of a variety of moderately effective chemotherapeutic agents the only modalities available for the treatment of small cell anaplastic lung cancer (SCALC) were the local modalities of surgery and radiotherapy. Trials performed with local modalities as the sole method of therapy were instrumental in establishing the virulent nature of this disease and its propensity for early dissemination. The 3–5-year survival rates observed in patients treated with surgery or radiotherapy alone ranged from zero to a maximum of 5% for patients with disease apparently limited to one hemithorax [1–5]. The lack of an association between the clinical stage of intrathoracic disease and survival led to an abandonment of the TNM staging system for SCALC [5]. Subsequently, the Veterans Administration Lung Cancer Study Group (VALSG) established a functional staging system which grouped patients into limited disease (confined to one hemithorax and/or the ipsilateral supraclavicular node) and extensive disease (outside the confines of limited disease) categories. The median survival times for placebo treated limited and extensive disease patients were 3 months and 6 weeks, respectively [6, 7].

In the same VALSG study, cyclophosphamide was shown to increase the median survival of extensive disease patients 2.5-fold [6]. Although this pioneering study was one of the first systematic studies to establish a role for chemotherapy, significant advances, particularly in limited disease patients, have occurred since that time to establish the pivotal, and potentially curative, role of aggressive combination chemotherapy in treating SCALC [8].

Since the discovery of the activity of cyclophosphamide, the activity of a variety of agents of different classes and toxicities has been described (Table 1) [9]. The potential exploitation of the modest activity of this group of

Greco, FA (ed), Biology and Management of Lung Cancer. ISBN 0-89838-554-7.
© *1983, Martinus Nijhoff Publishers, Boston. Printed in The Netherlands.*

Table 1. Single agents in small cell carcinoma.

Drug	No. patients	Response (%)	CR (%)
Cyclophosphamide	189	52 (28)	4
Adriamycin	36	11 (31)	–
Methotrexate	73	22 (30)	–
Vincristine	43	18 (42)	7
VP-16	167	75 (45)	9
CCNU	76	11 (14)	4
Hexamethylmelamine	69	21 (30)	7
HN$_2$	55	24 (44)	–

Adapted from Livingston [9].

single agents reached fruition with the design of several controlled randomized trials which established the superiority of combination chemotherapy over single agent treatment [10–12]. With this discovery, combinations of drugs were integrated into combined modality programs employing radiotherapy as the principal modality of local therapy. The use of aggressive combination chemotherapy combined with radiation therapy in limited disease patients led to an unquestionable increase in complete response, median survival and 2-year disease-free survival [8]. Certain studies have shown comparable results with the use of aggressive combination chemotherapy alone in limited disease patients [13–15].

At the present time, the value of 'sandwich' type radiation therapy, in which both the chemotherapy and radiation therapy doses and/or schedules are attenuated, is in question [16–18]. On the other hand, there is no study which has shown that aggressive combination chemotherapy is *superior* to a combined modality approach employing radiation therapy. In essence, then, the advances which have been made as a result of the application of aggressive combination chemotherapy, used alone or in conjunction with most radiation therapy schemes, have led to a plateau in the current expectations for long-term survival for patients with SCALC [19].

This impasse demands a thorough and honest reevaluation of where the last decade has taken us in the treatment of patients with SCALC and what the emphases and needs for the future must be. The obvious is to emphasize that the use of combination chemotherapy has increased the median survival of limited disease patients 4–5-fold with a 4–20-fold increase in 2-year survival. Alternatively, it could, and probably should, be emphasized that 50% of all limited disease patients die from uncontrolled disease within 12–16 months and approximately 80–90% of patients are dead from disease within 2 years.

Since the essence of SCALC is its disseminated nature, universally effective treatment will have to await the development of more effective drugs to be used in combination chemotherapy programs. Although it is not the subject of this report, an important area for reexamination should include a reevaluation of the format in which new agents are tested. New agents or programs are generally tested in refractory, poor performance status patients. In this setting a highly significant drug, VP-16-213, has yielded only a 10–15% objective response rate in our hands. Awaiting the discovery of more effective agents to be used in combination chemotherapy programs, another necessary approach to reconsider is the manner in which radiotherapy has been employed. The optimal radiation total dose, time/dose relationship and timing of combined modality treatment has been poorly explored [20]. Alternatives to 'sandwich' type radiation therapy include the use of simultaneous combination chemotherapy and radiation therapy [8, 21–24], and exploration of the role of superfractionation radiotherapy or the use of radiosensitizers.

Another area for reconsideration is the potential role of surgery in the combined modality management of SCALC. The subsequent discussion will relate to considerations relative to the history of the surgical treatment of SCALC, to the relevance, or irrelevance, of these observations in the current aggressive combination chemotherapy era, and to data generated at the SUNY Upstate Medical Center, Syracuse, New York testing the feasibility of using surgery as an adjuvant to combination chemotherapy for selected patients with limited disease.

2. BACKGROUND

During the late 1960s, the British Medical Research Council designed a study to test the efficacy of the two prime modalities available for the treatment of SCALC at that time, i.e. surgery and radiation therapy [2]. Patients with localized, potentially resectable disease, diagnosable by rigid bronchoscopy, were randomly allocated to surgical resection *versus* 'radical' radiation therapy. The results of this trial which showed that approximately 98% of patients died within 5 years proved that each of these modalities was incapable of significantly altering the outcome of SCALC. More germane to this discussion, this study was instrumental in eliminating surgery as a primary therapeutic modality for patients with SCALC, since the only survivors at 5 years were those patients who were treated with radiotherapy. Although this study was performed in the pre-chemotherapy era, it is still recognized as a major milestone which established, and continues to reinforce, the penultimate role of radiotherapy as the major local modality to be considered in the combined modality therapy of SCALC.

Mountain [5] has presented an extensive analysis of the results of a review of SCALC cases performed by the American Joint Committee for Staging and End Results Reporting from the pre-chemotherapy era. The results of this analysis showed that the T, N and M status of the tumor had no significant effect on survival when viewed as independent variables or when combined into stage groupings. Forty-one of 189 patients (22%) with disease limited to one hemothorax were deemed resectable for cure (Stage I - 15; Stage II - 5; Stage III - 21). The median survival of the resected patients was 5.0 months, with the longest survival being 39 months, as compared to the unresectable, and presumably more advanced, cases having a median survival of 5 months with the longest survival of 66 months. This study led to the abandonment of the TNM staging system for SCALC.

Other investigators have reported that long-term disease-free survival can be achieved in a certain small subset of patients who present with extremely limited disease [25, 20]. One of the first reports in this regard was presented by the Veterans Administration Surgical Adjuvant Group (VASAG) in a study addressing solitary pulmonary nodules. In this study a very small proportion of patients who had <6 cm lesions, outside of the diagnostic range of the rigid bronchoscope, were found to have histologically confirmed SCALC at thoracotomy [25]. Of the eleven resected patients fitting into this category, four (36%) survived 5 years. A more recent study has reported that approximately 40% of patients with Stage I disease survived 5 years after surgical resection [26]. Although this phenomenon has not been universally experienced [5], it does appear that a small proportion of an even smaller population of SCALC patients who present with Stage I disease might derive some benefit from surgical resection. With the advent of the flexible fiberoptic bronchoscope, it is almost certain that patients similar to those in the VASAG study with solitary, nondiagnosable pulmonary nodules might be diagnosable today. In light of the data mentioned above, it would not seem reasonable to summarily eliminate surgery as a prime local modality in a contemporary, prospectively diagnosed patient with a solitary pulmonary nodule.

It is difficult to estimate the exact proportion of patients with SCALC who would fit into this category; but it is quite small. Patients with Stage I disease represented 4% of the entire patient population and 9% of the limited disease population reported in the AJC analysis [5]. A similar small proportion of patients has been reported by Martini [27] and the Seattle Group [26]. Although 30–40% of these extremely limited disease patients may survive, it must be remembered that 60–70% develop disseminated metastases and die as a result.

During the conduct of an adjuvant chemotherapy trial employing cyclophosphamide reported by the VASAG a relatively small subset of patients

with Stage I and II SCALC were randomly allocated to adjunctive cyclophosphamide therapy. The patient numbers were too small to have a difference reach statistical significance, but it was shown that the survival in
the chemotherapy treated group was 16%, as compared to 4% in the surgery
alone group [28]. Similarly, the Austrian Group has reported comparable
data using a moderately toxic combination of drugs including cyclophosphamide, 5-fluorouracil, vinblastine and methotrexate [29]. No large study,
to date, has compared the use of currently accepted, aggressive combination
chemotherapy to local therapy alone in such patients.

As mentioned before, the significant advances which have been made
over the last several years have resulted from the development of aggressive
combination chemotherapy programs. The systematic integration of a local
modality into the therapeutic research scheme has relied, virtually exclusively, on radiation therapy. The use of attenuated doses and/or schedules
of each modality has led to a question as to whether adding the local component, embodied by radiation therapy as employed in most studies, offers
any substantial benefit over chemotherapy alone. This question has, to a
certain extent, blurred the issue of the need to control the *entire* disease
process, including both the *primary tumor* and subclinical metastases in
limited disease patients. Without control of the entire disease process, cure
cannot be achieved.

There is substantial evidence which indicates that current modalities and
therapeutic programs are incapable of controlling the primary site of bulk
disease within the chest. As with many other malignancies, the site of bulk
disease is a major site of initial relapse. The conventional approach to
defining complete remission in limited disease patients relies primarily on
the chest radiograph. Complete resolution of previous intrathoracic disease
occurs in about 50-60% of limited disease patients [8, 30]. Ihde [31] has
presented data comparing the appearance of the chest radiograph to the
results of serial fiberoptic bronchoscopy and bronchoscopic biopsy. Eighty-
one procedures were performed in 38 patients who had achieved complete
radiographic response of the primary tumor. Bronchoscopically documented
abnormalities were present in 36%. At twelve weeks, intrathoracic relapse
occurred in 75% of the complete responding patients with bronchoscopic
abnormalities, as opposed to 19% in those in whom no bronchoscopic
abnormalities were detected. Overall 35% of complete responding patients
relapsed within the chest, as well as 47% of partial, or nonresponding
patients.

It is difficult to cull from the literature the precise incidence of initial
failure in the chest in limited disease patients. This difficulty relates to there
not being any uniform method of data reporting adhered to by various
authors. Table 2 presents data from 10 combined modality studies [16, 32-

Table 2. Chest relapse in responding limited disease patients[a].

Investigator	Treatment regimen	Number of responding patients	% with chest relapse (No.)			Relapse pattern % chest only
			All patients	CR only	PR only	
Livingston et al. [32]	CAV × 3 − 2000r/10 − 2 wk 1500/5-CAV	36	67 (24)	61 (13/21)	73 (11/15)	100 (24/24)
Mira and Livingston [33]	As above	17	41 ((7))	—	—	100 (7/7)
Feld [34]	CAV × 3-2500r/10-CPM	40	50 (20)	—	—	45 (9/20)
Fox et al. [16, 35]	CAV × 3-4000r/20-CAV	28	32 (9)	—	—	100 (9/9)
Johnson et al. [36]	CAV + various RT	13[c]	77 (10)	77 (10/13)		100 (10/10)
Holoye et al. [37]	CV-3000r/10-4 wk-3000r/10CV	16	6 (1)	—	—	100 (1/1)
McMahon et al. [38]	AC-3000r/10 or 4000-4500r/30-55-AC-CMV	10	60 (6)	—	—	100 (6/6)
Levitt et al. [39]	2000r/5-2000r/5-CCV-AV	15	53 (8)	62 (5/8)	43 (3/7)	100 (8/8)
Abeloff et al. [40]	BOMPZ-3500-4000r/15-20-BOMPZ	8	35 (3)	60 (3/5)	—	20 (1/5)
Totals		183	47 (88)	67 (31/47)	63 (14/22)	85 (75/88)

[a] Combined modality studies in which initial relapse is described for responding patients either as a group or stratified by response parameter.

[b] One patient developed metastatic disease within one month.

[c] Only CR reported.

40] in which the data were reported in such a manner that an analysis of the percentage of patients in whom initial primary site relapse could be established. The analysis is restricted to the relapse pattern in responding patients, and, as a result, it probably significantly underestimates the real importance of the problem. It can be seen that overall 47% of responding patients relapsed within the chest. Of these cases, it appears that 88% occur as the sole, initial site of relapse without evidence of concomitant relapse in other disease sites. Data were available in only 25% (47/183) of the cases reviewed to establish the initial site of relapse in complete responding patients. In two thirds of these cases recurrence within the chest occurred as the initial site of relapse. It is the impression of many investigators that local relapse is only a harbinger of rapid, disseminated relapse. Possibly because of reporting deficiencies, this is not the impression that one obtains from the literature. Only one paper, by Feld [34], defined the temporal relationship between initial chest relapse and the subsequent relapse pattern. In this study 20 patients developed chest relapse. Nine of 20 patients (45%) developed relapse in the primary site *only* prior to death; 1/20 (5%) relapsed outside the chest within one month, and 10/20 (50%) patients subsequently developed disseminated disease greater than one month after local relapse had occurred. In summary, local relapse with or without subsequent disseminated relapse is a major problem with contemporary combined modality programs.

Currently, it is impossible to define the relationship between a chronically uncontrolled primary tumor and the subsequent development of disseminated disease. The impact of the lack of local control on survival and/or the subsequent clinical course of the disease has only been rarely addressed. Mira and Livingston [33] have indicated that complications relating to uncontrolled chest disease accounted for 53% (9/17) of the deaths in their limited disease patients, including complications arising from primary chest recurrences, infection, hemoptysis and 'other' chest problems. Similarly, Gilby *et al.* [41] estimated that recurrence of the primary tumor represented the 'predominant' cause of death in 41% of their cases. Thus, it is quite possible that in addition to representing a major cause of primary treatment failure, uncontrolled chest disease may represent a substantial cause of death in limited disease patients.

In light of the foregoing discussion, the contemporary relevance of the British Medical Research Council study which led to the abandonment of surgery as a primary therapeutic modality must be questioned. This study was performed prior to the availability of chemotherapeutic agents with the potential of treating, and in some instances, eradicating subclinical, metastatic disease. The conclusion of the study relative to the lack of a considered role for surgery was pertinent to its time, but it is quite questionable whether the current status of therapy available for patients with SCALC justifies the adherence to this conclusion at the present time.

3. SUNY UPSTATE MEDICAL CENTER, ADJUVANT SURGERY TRIAL

We decided to launch a trial to establish the feasibility of employing surgery as the primary local modality for selected patients with SCALC as a result of several factors. First, as mentioned above, local relapse in the primary site is a major problem encountered with current combined modality approaches. In launching the trial the possibility that this problem might be a trivial one was well appreciated, i.e. that if primary site relapse were eliminated, disseminated relapse might become the predominant mode of relapse for the majority of patients. Secondly, thirty-eight percent of our long-term survivors, as reported by Ginsberg et al. [42] received surgery as an integral part of their primary treatment program. Thirdly, we had the cooperation and intense interest of our thoracic surgeons in evaluating this approach spearheaded by Dr John J. Meyer who aptly described our joint experience with a patient who had a T_2N_1 tumor diagnosed at thoracotomy who was purposely not resected, and who ultimately died of uncontrolled intrathoracic disease without demonstrable metastasis at autopsy, after a complete remission for 18 months [42]. Lastly, surgery could potentially induce a rapid, complete clinical remission with little myelosuppressive or immunosuppressive expense.

For small cell lung cancer, it is generally accepted that the potential role for surgery should be viewed as an adjuvant to chemotherapy, the pivotal modality of therapy. The consideration of which modality is adjunctive to the other is, to a certain extent, as much a function of medical history as it is of biology. For instance, breast cancer patients with 4 or more positive axillary lymph nodes have a median survival of approximately 18 months, and 85% die from disseminated disease within 5 years. Aggressive adjuvant chemotherapy has significantly decreased the relapse rate and increased the survival rate and possibility for cure. Because the therapeutic history of breast cancer has been steeped in surgical management for almost a century, chemotherapy is viewed as an adjuvant to surgery, when, in fact, the removal of bulk disease in the primary and regional site could be more appropriately viewed as an adjunct to systemic therapy necessary for control of the disseminated micrometastatic disease to which 85% of the patients succumb. In any case, it would seem appropriate to view surgery as an adjuvant to chemotherapy for SCALC considering its clinical course and history.

The adjuvant surgery study was designed to test the feasibility of employing surgery as an integral part of a program to rapidly induce complete clinical remission. To this end patients with markedly limited lesions (Stage I–II) receive immediate surgery followed by adjunctive chemotherapy within 3–4 weeks for 1 year. Patients with more advanced lesions (ipsilateral T_3 and/or N_2 disease) are treated with 2–4 cycles of chemotherapy followed by surgery with the intent to remove all gross disease. In the latter group, the timing of surgery was based upon the shape of the survival curve for complete responders obtained at our institution prior to the initiation of the adjuvant surgery trial. As with most studies in the literature, patients remained in complete remission for approximately 6 months, prior to developing a linear decrease in disease control and survival [43]. An alternative approach would have been to delay surgery for several months and employ it as a method of local consolidation in confirmed chemotherapy complete responders. We felt that this approach was somewhat less attractive since: (1) chemotherapy is only capable of eradicating the total disease process in 10–20% of patients; (2) in spite of an apparent complete clinical remission at least 1/3 of patients would have persistently uncontrolled local disease; and (3) the presence of an uncontrolled primary tumor might allow for the continued dissemination of drug-resistant cells. The general scheme of the study is presented in Table 3.

Eligibility criteria currently include that: the disease be ipsilateral as confirmed by mediastinoscopy; the patient have adequate pulmonary reserve to tolerate a pneumonectomy if necessary ($FEV_1 > 1.6$ L, $pCO_2 < 42$ mmHg) and have no medical contraindication to surgery or the use of adriamycin; although phrenic or recurrent laryngeal nerve involvement, or minimal superior vena caval obstruction did not disqualify patients, patients could not have evidence for severe superior vena caval obstruction involvement of major vessels which precluded complete removal of the primary or regional disease, or a malignant pleural effusion. Since this was a feasibility study the aforementioned criteria, particularly with regard to the patient's pulmonary status and the preoperative response to chemotherapy evolved during the course of the trial, as will be discussed below.

Table 3. General plan of therapy.

Stage I + II	Surgery → Chemo
Stage III	Chemo → Surgery
Eligibility	1. No medical contraindicators
	2. No prior CHF
	3. Ipsilateral T_3 or N_2 only
	4. No severe SVC, direct extension, malignant pleural effusion
	5. Negative metastatic evaluation

Table 4

Total No. patients	24
Male: Female	14:10
Mean age	60

TNM stage:

I	$T_{1-2} N_{0-1}$	–	6
II	$T_2 N_1$	–	3
III	T_3 and/or N_2	–	15
	$T_3 N_0$	–	2
	$T_1 N_2$	–	1
	$T_2 N_2$	–	8
	$T_3 N_2$	–	4

Chemotherapy programs[a]

CCV^b	–	8
CAVE	–	16

Planned treatment scheme

Surgery – Chemotherapy	9
Chemotherapy – Surgery	15

[a] See text.
[b] One patient received adriamycin (CCVAV); three patients received radiation therapy.

The pretreatment evaluation included a complete history and physical examination; pulmonary function tests including spirometry and arterial blood gases; bronchoscopy and mediastinoscopy; routine laboratory work including a complete blood count, platelet count, electrolytes, liver and renal function tests; radionuclide scans of the bone and liver; CAT scan of the brain; and bilateral bone marrow aspirate and biopsies. Although a CAT scan of the chest was not required most patients received a chest CAT scan at some time prior to surgery.

The current pre- and/or postoperative chemotherapeutic program employs CAVE chemotherapy (cyclophosphamide 1.0 gm/M^2 q 3 weeks; adriamycin 35 mg/M^2 q 3 weeks; vincristine 2.0 mg weekly $\times$ 6, then q 3 weeks, and etoposide 50 mg/M^2/d $\times$ 5 q 3 weeks). Earlier patients generally received a combination of CCNU, cyclophosphamide and vincristine (CCV). Chemotherapy is currently administered for one year, with all patients receiving elective cranial irradiation.

To date 24 patients have been considered for the combined modality program. The pertinent patient-related characteristics are presented in Table 4. All patients had a performance status of 0–1. Five of the nine patients who presented with Stage I–II disease had histologically or cytologically confirmed preoperative diagnoses of SCALC.

Table 5 describes the programmatic results obtained in these 24 patients. One patient is currently undergoing preoperative chemotherapy and is too

Table 5

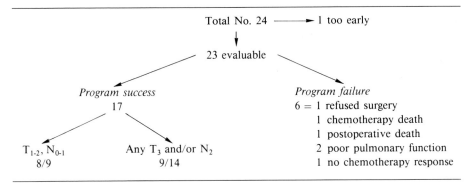

Total No. 24 ⟶ 1 too early

23 evaluable

Program success
17

Program failure
6 = 1 refused surgery
1 chemotherapy death
1 postoperative death
2 poor pulmonary function
1 no chemotherapy response

T_{1-2}, N_{0-1}
8/9

Any T_3 and/or N_2
9/14

---

early to evaluate. Seventeen patients (74%) have undergone the combined modality program including surgery and chemotherapy and are termed a 'program success'. The reasons for 'program failure' are outlined in Table 6. One patient with T_2N_2 disease refused surgery after a response to induction chemotherapy. Two treatment-related deaths have occurred. One patient with a T_2N_0 tumor died during surgical convalescence from a massive pulmonary embolus. The second patient (T_2N_2) died from the result of a destructive thrombocytopenia, compounded by the effects of chemotherapy. Both patients had a single site of documented metastatic disease at autopsy in the retroperitoneum and liver, respectively. Two patients (1, T_3N_2; 1, T_2N_2) had persistently poor pulmonary function which precluded pneumonectomy after chemotherapy response. In both instances the patients had significant lobar collapse and marginal pulmonary functions prior to induction chemotherapy. At the time of their presentation, it was anticipated that if a significant response to chemotherapy occurred, concomitant improvement in pulmonary function might allow an attempt at appropriate surgical resection. Although a significant chemotherapy response occurred in both patients, persistent pulmonary function abnormalities precluded complete surgical resection in both. Since this experience, the decision to enter a Stage III disease patient is based solely on the prechemotherapy pulmonary function status. Finally, one patient with a Pancoast syndrome did not respond to preoperative chemotherapy. As will be discussed below, our experience prior to entering this patient indicated that chemotherapy nonresponders rapidly succumb to their disease. Presently, only patients who experience at least a partial remission are considered for surgery. All four patients who did not receive surgery received chemotherapy alone or in combination with radiotherapy. Two of these four patients (1 CR, 1 NR) are dead at 11 and 14 months, respectively; one complete responding patient is alive at 14 months

Table 6

Patient No.	TNM[a] stage	Treatment scheme	Type of surgery[c]	Survival	Remarks[d]
1	T_2N_2	CCV/RT – S	L	8	no response to chemotherapy
2	T_3N_2	CCV/RT – S	P	10	no response to chemotherapy, widespread disease at autopsy
3	T_2N_2	CAVE – S	P	7+	NED
4	T_2N_2[b]	CAVE – S	P	12+	NED
5	T_2N_2	CAVE – S	P	13+	NED
6	T_2N_0	S – CAVE	P	15	died with spinal cord and liver metastasis
7	T_2N_2	CAVE – S	L	17	died with meningeal disease only
8	T_1N_0	S – CAVE	L	19+	NED
9	T_3N_3	CAVE – S	P	23+	NED
10	T_2N_0	S CAVE	S	24+	NED
11	T_3N_0	CAVE – S	P	34+	NED
12	T_1N_2	CCV – S	L	34	relapsed at 24 months with liver and porta hepatitis metastasis; responded to VP-16 DDP; no local disease at autopsy
13	T_2N_0	S – CCV	L	35+	NED
14	T_1N_0	S – CCV	L	49+	NED
15	T_2N_1	S – CCV-AV	L	50	died from disseminated prostate CA; no SCALC at autopsy
16	T_2N_1	S – CCV	L	54+	NED
17	T_2N_1	S – CCV/RT	L	76+	NED

[a] At the time of surgery for T_{1-2}, N_{0-1}; at the time of chemotherapy for all others.
[b] L = lobectomy; P = pneumectomy; S = segmentectomy.
[d] NED = currently disease-free.
[b] Patient refused further chemotherapy after 6 months.

with recurrence in the chest and contralateral supraclavicular node, and one patient is alive in continuing complete remission at 14 months.

The status of the 17 patients who received surgery and chemotherapy is presented in Table 6. Currently 11 patients are alive and disease-free at a median time of 24+ months (range 7+–76+ months). Six deaths have recurred, with one of the six patients having died from disseminated prostatic carcinoma, with no SCALC apparent at autopsy. Patients Nos. 1 and 2 illustrate the point that was mentioned above regarding the preoperative response to chemotherapy. Both patients were entered during the initial phase of the study, and neither responded to CCV chemotherapy. After considerable discussion, radiation therapy was employed, with apparent response of the intrathoracic disease. In spite of this response the patients rapidly succumbed, presumably because their disease was chemotherapy unresponsive. Autopsies have been performed in 4 of the 6 patients who have died. No patient has had evidence of residual intrathoracic disease. Of the 5 patients who have died from SCALC, 3 developed widespread metastases; one patient died from meningeal disease which occurred directly in the radiation therapy portal, with no other demonstrable tumor at autopsy; and the precise pattern of disease spread at the time of death is unknown in the final patient.

Table 7 shows the clinical chemotherapy response compared to the preoperative and postoperative TNM stage in patients who were treated with chemotherapy prior to surgery. Only one patient had no histologically demonstrable disease at the time of surgery. In addition only an occasional patient had 'downstaging' of the disease after chemotherapy. It is difficult to interpret the significance of these data since the purpose of therapy was not to treat to maximal response, i.e. clinical complete remission, but rather to relatively rapidly perform surgery as an integral part of induction therapy. In any case, only 1/9 patients had a complete response to chemotherapy on a histologic basis. Of interest is Case No. 4 (Table 7) who received 2 cycles (6 weeks) of CAVE chemotherapy prior to surgical resection. Preoperatively, SCALC was demonstrated on both the bronchoscopic and mediastinoscopic biopsies. In the operative specimen, cells resembling the initial biopsy were

Table 7. Clinical chemotherapy response compared to re- and postoperative TNM stage.

Patient No.[a]	AJC stage preoperative	Clinical response	AJC stage postoperative
9	T_3N_0	CR	T_0N_0
11	T_3N_0	PR	T_1N_1
12	T_1N_2	PR	T_1N_2
7	T_2N_2	TR	T_2N_2
5	T_2N_2	PR	T_2N_2
4	T_2N_2	PR	T_2N_2
3	T_2N_2	PR	T_2N_2
2	T_2N_2	NR	T_2N_2[b]
1	T_3N_2	NR	T_2N_0[b]

[a] See Table 7 for corresponding data.
[b] Had radiotherapy after chemotherapy nonresponse.

present within a marked fibrotic reaction at the primary site, and papillary adenocarcinoma was in the tissue obtained at the mediastinal node dissection. The histological appearance of the specimens obtained in this study will be the subject of another report. Briefly, the histologic appearance of tumor in the resected specimen has ranged from no demonstrable alteration in cellular appearance, to marked ballooning and distortion of cells, to, in one case, massive necrosis without evident tumor. In general, the resected specimens contain a significant amount of necrosis, and acute and chronic inflammation in the surrounding lung tissue.

The type of operation performed is to a great extent dependent upon the stage of the primary tumor. The timing of surgery in Stage III patients is decided jointly by the medical oncologist and surgeon. The majority of patients with T_3 and/or N_2 disease require pneumonectomy and mediastinal node dissection, while most patients presenting with T_{1-2}, N_{0-1} disease require only lobectomy. The chemotherapy toxicities are similar to those anticipated and described by others who have employed similar regimens [13]. The only unusual constitutional toxicity has been the development of marked weight loss (> 10 % body weight) in 3 Stage III patients subsequent to surgery which required an aggressive enteral hyperalimentation in one patient. This patient refused chemotherapy at 5 months, and is in a continuing complete remission at 12+ months.

4. DISCUSSION

The nature of SCALC led to the abandonment of surgery as a primary tool in the therapeutic management of SCALC. This approach was justifiable in the prechemotherapeutic era since less morbidity and comparably poor results could be obtained with radiation therapy alone. The advent of aggressive combination chemotherapy has led to significant improvement in the median survival of patients with limited disease as well as to the possibility for long-term disease-free survival. Yet, the majority of patients die from their disease within 12–16 months, and 80–90 % are dead, in spite of an initial response to chemotherapy, within 2 years. Relapse in the chest is a major component of relapse from complete and partial remission, and it may, in fact be a major cause of death in limited disease patients. These factors led us to reconsider the role of surgery as a primary modality in the therapeutic research strategy for selected limited disease patients.

The results of our study to date indicate that, at least, this combined modality approach is feasible in not only patients with Stage I–II disease, but also in selected patients with Stage III disease. It should be emphasized that in our study the anatomic basis for patient selection resided in the application of the TNM staging system as suggested by the American Joint Committee for Staging and End Results reporting. It is clear that if the application of surgery as a potential local modality is to be pursued the TNM staging system must be reintroduced into the clinicopathologic staging system for SCALC. This will provide a tool for the comparison of results from study to study, and also provide a precise definition for patient selection in comparative trials. Since patient selection is a major component of our program, it is extremely unfortunate that no contemporary control group, as defined by the TNM system, is available to us for comparison. Although our results appear strikingly different from those reported by Mountain [5], a valid comparison cannot be made because of the vast differences in the presurgical evaluation of contemporarily staged limited disease patients. To these ends, one of the recommendations emanating from a recent international consensus meeting held at Ashford Castle, Ireland will be to reinstitute the TNM staging system for this disease.

In addition to being a feasible approach the preliminary results of our study are somewhat encouraging. Eight patients, representing 35% of those considered for the program and 47% of those who actually received surgery,

Table 8. Small cell anaplastic lung cancer long-term (≥ 24 months) survival, SUNY Upstate Medical Center.

| No. | Stage | Chemotherapy | | Survival (months) | Remarks[a] |
		Radiotherapy	Surgery		
1	III	–	+	24	NED
2	I	–	+	24	NED
3	III	–	+	34	DOD
4	III	–	+	34	NED
5	II	–	+	35	NED
6	Lim	+	–	44	NED
7	I	–	+	49	NED
8	II	–	+	50	DOC
9	II	–	+	54	NED
10	Lim	+	–	60	DOD[b]
11	Lim	+	–	64	NED
12	Lim	+	–	68	NED
13	Lim	+	–	69	NED
14	II	+	+	76	NED
15	Ext	–	–	31	NED
16	Ext	+	–	76	NED

[a] DOD = died of disease; DOC = died of other causes.
[b] Developed adenocarcinoma in primary site with widespread metastases.

survived ≥24 months. Only one of these patients has relapsed and died from SCALC. Of the remaining 9 patients who have survived less than 24 months, 5 are alive and disease-free at 23+, 19+, 13+, 12+ and 7+ months, respectively. The preliminary results are particularly striking in the patients who presented with Stage I–II disease in which 7 of 9 patients (78%), including the patient who died postoperatively, are alive and disease-free with a median survival of 35+ months. A composite of the long-term (>24 months) survival experience at the SUNY Upstate Medical Center is presented in Table 8. It can be seen that two thirds of our 14 limited disease patients who survived for ≥24 months had surgery as a primary component of their treatment. Since it is well established that combination chemotherapy used alone, or in conjunction with radiotherapy, can cure patients (33% of our limited disease long-term survivors) it is impossible to be certain whether this overrepresentation of surgically treated cases is a function of our interest in this modality or its therapeutic power when used together with combination chemotherapy.

In addition to the available survival data the patterns of relapse and autopsy data are of particular interest. Complete clinical and/or autopsy data relating to relapse is available in 5 of the 6 patients who have died, 4 of whom received post-mortem examinations. No patient had evidence of relapse within the primary site or chest. Central nervous system relapse was a primary component of relapse in 2 of the 4 patients who survived greater than one year, and was the sole site of relapse and cause of death in one of these patients. Therefore, to date it appears that initial relapse within the primary site has been virtually eliminated with this approach.

The availability of tissue from preoperative and surgical specimens may also provide useful information concerning the biology of SCALC in the future. It is of interest that one of our patients had a 'shift' in the pattern of disease from intermediate SCALC to papillary adenocarcinoma after only 2 cycles of chemotherapy. Although this is a well-described phenomenon, the rapidity with which this occurred in our case was striking. The availability of serum-free, conditioned media [45], which has greatly increased the ability to culture and clone SCALC, will hopefully provide insights into the biology of the disease, particularly with regard to drug resistance, when these techniques are successfully integrated into programs in which surgically derived tissue is available.

5. SUMMARY AND CONCLUSIONS

It appears that surgery can be effectively incorporated into the therapeutic research strategy for selected patients with SCALC. Our preliminary data indicate that local control can be achieved, and, as a result, that a major therapeutic problem, i.e. initial relapse in the primary site, can be effectively addressed. Whether our encouraging results will be sustained in larger trials is unknown, as is the relative value of surgery compared to more conventional approaches in similarly selected and staged patients.

This relative question can only be addressed by properly designed and executed Phase III trials with particular attention to selected patients with ipsilateral Stage III disease. Patients with Stage I and II disease represent a different problem, since there are probably only 1–1.5 thousand cases in the whole nation per year. Our average case accrual for this group is only 1.4/year. In this group we may have to consider 'playing the winner' short of instituting a nationwide trial. Most patients in this category were able to be completely resected with lobectomy as the most common operative procedure. But it is clear that even with the best of statistics 60–70% of these patients will succumb to metastatic disease. A reasonable approach to this group would be to consider surgery plus aggressive combination chemotherapy as the primary mode of therapy at the present time.

Until truly effective chemotherapeutic agents become available, the need for controlling the bulk disease site in limited disease patients will remain to be a significant therapeutic problem. Awaiting the development of such agents, no modality which has the potential of addressing this important problem should be excluded from the therapeutic research strategy.

REFERENCES

1. Bergsagel D, Jenkins R, Pringle J, et al.: Lung cancer: clinical trial of radiotherapy alone versus radiotherapy plus cyclophosphamide. Cancer 30:621–727, 1972.
2. Fox W, Scadding JG: Medical Research Council comparative trial of surgery and radiotherapy for the primary treatment of small celled or oat cell carcinoma of the bronchus. Ten year follow-up. Lancet 2:63–65, 1973.
3. Laing AH, Berry RJ, Newman CR: Treatment of small cell carcinoma of the bronchus. Lancet 1:129–132, 1975.
4. Lee RE, Carr DT, Childs DS: Comparison of split course radiation therapy and continuous radiation therapy for unresectable bronchogenic carcinoma: 5 year results. Am J Roentgenol Radium Ther Nuc Med 126:116–122, 1976.
5. Mountain CF: Clinical biology of small cell lung cancer: Relationship to surgical therapy. Sem Oncol 5:272–279, 1978.
6. Green RA, Hymphrey E, Close HM, et al.: Alkylating agents in bronchogenic carcinoma. Am J Med 46:516–525, 1969.
7. Zelen M: Keynote address on biostatistics and data retrieval. Cancer Chemother Rep 4:31–42, 1973.
8. Oldham RK, Greco FA, Einhorn LH, et al.: Preliminary results of a randomized trial to evaluate the role of radiotherapy in the combined modality therapy of limited stage small cell lung cancer. Proc Amer Soc Clin Oncol 22:505, 1981.

9. Livingston RB: Treatment of small cell carcinoma: Evolution and future direction. Sem Oncol 5:299–308, 1978.
10. Alberto P, Brunner KW, Martz G, et al.: Treatment of bronchogenic carcinoma with simultaneous or sequential combination chemotherapy, including methotrexate, cyclophosphamide, procarbazine and vincristine. Cancer 38:2208–2216, 1976.
11. Edmonson JH, Lagakos SS, Selawry OS, et al.: Cyclophosphamide plus CCNU compared to cyclophosphamide alone in the treatment of small cell and adenocarcinoma of the lung. Cancer Treat Rep 60:925–932, 1976.
12. Lowenbraun S, Bertolucci A, Smalley RV, et al.: The superiority of combination chemotherapy over single agent chemotherapy in small cell lung cancer. Cancer 44:406–413, 1979.
13. Aisner J, Whitacre M, Van Echo DA, et al.: Alternating noncrossresistant combination chemotherapy for small cell carcinoma of the lung. Proc Am Assoc Cancer Res 21:453, 1980.
14. Cohen MH, Creaven PI, Fosseick BE, et al.: Intensive chemotherapy of small cell bronchogenic carcinoma. Cancer Treat Rep 349–354, 1979.
15. Israel L, DiPierre A, Choffel C: Immunochemotherapy in 34 cases of oat cell carcinoma of the lung with 19 complete responses. Cancer Treat Rep 61:343–347, 1977.
16. Fox RM, Tattersall MHN, Woods RL: Radiation therapy as an adjuvant in small cell lung cancer treated by combination chemotherapy: A randomized study. Proc Amer Soc Clin Oncol 22:502, 1981.
17. Hansen HH, Dombernowsky P, Hansen HS, Rorth M: Chemotherapy *versus* chemotherapy plus radiotherapy in regional small cell carcinoma of the lung – a randomized trial. Proc Am Assoc Cancer Res 20:277, 1979.
18. Stevens E, Einhorn L, Rohn R: Treatment of limited small cell lung cancer. Proc Am Assoc Cancer Res 20:435, 1979.
19. Cohen MH: Small cell lung cancer: restained optimism. Int J Radiat Oncol Biol Phys 6:1119–1120, 1980.
20. Salazar OM, Creech RH: The state of the art: Toward defining the role of radiation therapy in the management of small cell lung cancer. Int. J Radiat Oncol Biol Phys 6: 1103–1117, 1977.
21. Catane R, Lichter A, Lee J, et al.: Small cell lung cancer. Analysis of treatment factors contributing to prolonged survival. Cancer 48:1936–1943, 1981.
22. Cohen MH, Lichter AS, Bunn PA, Glatstein ES, et al.: Chemotherapy-radiation therapy (CT-RT) *versus* chemotherapy (CT) in limited small cell lung cancer (SCLC). Proc Am Assoc Cancer Res 21:448, 1980.
23. Greco FA, Richardson RL, Sulman SF, et al.: Therapy of oat cell carcinoma of the lung: complete remissions, acceptable complications and improved survival. Br Med J 2:10–11, 1978.
24. Perry CD, Eaton WL, Comis RL, et al.: Simultaneous radiation therapy and chemotherapy in limited small cell cancer of the lung: a pilot study. Proc Amer Soc Clinical Oncol 22:503, 1981.
25. Higgins CA, Shields TW, Keehn RJ: The solitary pulmonary nodule. Ten year follow-up of Veterans Administration – Armed Forces cooperative study. Arch Surg 110:570–575, 1975.
26. Wright P, Shulman S, Davis S, et al.: Unexpectedly favorable survival without intensive combination chemotherapy in patients with small cell lung cancer. Proc Amer Soc Clin Oncol 22:493, 1981.
27. Martini N, Wittes R, Hilaris BS, et al.: Oat cell carcinoma of the lung. Clin Bull 5:144–148, 1975.

28. Shields TW: Status report of adjuvant cancer chemotherapy trials in the treatment of bronchial carcinoma. Cancer Chemother Rep 4: 119–124, 1973.
29. Karrer K: Adjuvant chemotherapy of post surgical minimal residual bronchial carcinomas. Recent Results Cancer Res 68:246–259, 1979.
30. Bunn PA, Cohen MH, Ihde DC, et al.: Advances in small cell bronchogenic carcinoma. Cancer Treat Rep 61:333–342, 1977.
31. Ihde DC, Cohen MH, Bernaton AM, Matthews MJ, et al.: Serial fiberoptic bronchoscopy during chemotherapy for small cell carcinoma of the lung. Early detection of patients at high risk for relapse. Chest 74:531–536, 1978.
32. Livingston RB, Moore TN, Helibrun L, et al.: Small cell carcinoma of the lung: combined chemotherapy and radiation: a Southwest Oncology Group Study. Ann Intern Med 88:194–199, 1978.
33. Mira JG, Livingston RB: Evaluation and radiotherapy implications of chest relapse patterns in small cell lung carcinoma treated with radiotherapy – chemotherapy: study of 34 cases and review of the literature. Cancer 46:2557–2565, 1980.
34. Feld R: Complications in the treatment of small cell carcinoma of the lung. Cancer Treat Rev 8:5–26, 1981.
35. Fox RM, Woods RL, Brodie GN, Tattersall MH: A randomized study: small cell anaplastic lung cancer treated by combination chemotherapy and adjuvant radiotherapy. Int J Radiat Oncol Biol Phys 6:1083–1085, 1980.
36. Johnson RE, Brereton HD, Kent CH: Total therapy for small cell carcinoma of the lung. Ann Thorac Surg 25:510–515, 1978.
37. Holoye PY, Samuels ML, Lanzalotti VJ, et al.: Combination chemotherapy and radiotherapy for small cell carcinoma. JAMA 237:1221–1224, 1977.
38. McMahon LA, Herman TS, Manning MR, Dean JC: Patterns of relapse in patients with small cell carcinoma of the lung treated with adriamycin-cyclophosphamide chemotherapy and radiation therapy. Cancer Treat Rep 63:359–362, 1979.
39. Levitt M, Meikle A, Murray N, Weinerman B: Oat cell carcinoma of the lung. CNS metastasis in spite of prophylactic brain irradiation. Cancer Treat Rep 62:131–133, 1978.
40. Abeloff MD, Ettinger DS, Baylin SB, Hazra T: Management of small cell carcinoma of the lung: Therapy, staging and biochemical markers. Cancer 38:1394–1401, 1976.
41. Gilby ED, Bondy PK, Morgan RL, et al.: Combination chemotherapy for small cell carcinoma of the lung. Cancer 39:1959–1960, 1977.
42. Ginsberg SJ, Comis RL, Gottlieb AJ: Long-term survivorship in small cell anaplastic lung carcinoma. Cancer Treat Rep 63:1347–1349, 1979.
43. Meyer JA, Comis RL, Ginsberg SJ, et al.: Selective surgical resection in small cell carcinoma of the lung. J Thoracic Cardiovasc Surg 77:243–248, 1979.
44. King G, Comis RL, Ginsberg S, et al.: Combination multiple chemotherapy and radiotherapy in small cell carcinoma of the lung. Radiology 125:529–530, 1977.
45. Gazdar A, Carney DN, Russell EK, et al.: Establishment of continuous, clonable cultures of small cell carcinoma of the lung which have amine precursor uptake and decarboxylation properties. Cancer Res 40: 3502–3507, 1980.

11. Chemotherapy and Radiation Therapy of Non-Small Cell Lung Carcinoma

KENNETH R. HANDE and ARNOLD W. MALCOLM

1. INTRODUCTION

Carcinoma of the lung remains the leading cause of death due to malignant disease in the United States, and is rapidly becoming the leading cause of cancer death in women [1]. Although surgical therapy of non-small cell lung cancers has improved during the past two decades, the overall results remain discouraging. The limited efficacy of surgical therapy has led to exploration of other treatment modalities such as radiation or chemotherapy either alone or in combination with surgery, particularly for the two thirds of the patients who present with advanced disease and for those in whom the presence of associated disease renders resection too hazardous. This chapter will attempt to review the present limitations and usefulness of radiation therapy and chemotherapy in the treatment of non-small cell lung cancer.

2. RADIATION THERAPY

Like surgery, irradiation is local treatment for disease which in many cases is or becomes rapidly systemic. Irradiation has been utilized in several ways in the therapy of non-small cell carcinoma (i.e., alone, postoperatively, preoperatively, in combination with chemotherapy, and palliatively). Reasonable evidence exists that radiation can sterilize non-small cell lung cancers. Four series [2–5] evaluating preoperative irradiation (usually 5000–6000 rads) as an adjunct to surgery, have demonstrated that 40% of cases irradiated and subsequently resected have no evidence of viable tumor in the specimen (Table 1). Similarly, in a study of 60 autopsies of patients with inoperable cancer treated with megavoltage irradiation (4800–6200 rads), no cancer was found in the irradiated field in 18 (30%), small nests of nests

Greco, FA (ed), Biology and Management of Lung Cancer. ISBN 0-89838-554-7.
© *1983, Martinus Nijhoff Publishers, Boston. Printed in The Netherlands.*

Table 1. Cases treated with preoperative irradiation and subsequent resection.

Reference	Dose (rads)	Number of case	No evidence of tumor in resected specimen
Bloedorn *et al.* [2]	5,500–6,000	17	9
Bromley and Szur [3]	3,700–6,000	11	5
Hellman *et al.* [4]	5,500–6,000	24	19
Shields [5]	4,000–5,000	84	23
Total		137	56 (41%)

of carcinoma cells admixed with fibrosis or extensive necrosis in another 20 (33%), and carcinoma appearing fully viable in only 22 (37%) [6]. In this study, 8 of the 18 patients in whom local sterilization appeared to have been achieved, died of distant metastases. These studies suggest that it is possible to achieve local sterilization of tumor by irradiation in a significant proportion of cases.

2.1. Radiation therapy as an adjunct to surgery

2.1.1. Preoperative irradiation. As mentioned in the previous section, preoperative irradiation can achieve sterilization of tumor prior to surgery. Several lines of evidence indicate that operations thought to have been complete and curative at the time of surgery are often associated with residual disease. Higgins [7] found that 26% of patients dying within 30 days of what was believed to be a complete resection had residual disease at postmortem examination. Other studies have found a 15% incidence of microscopic tumor demonstrable in the bronchial stump and a 40% incidence of recurrent local disease in patients autopsied after curative resection. The presence or absence of mediastinal node involvement (an area where irradiation can potentially sterilize tumor) also predicts for surgical cure [8]. A basic rationale for the use of preoperative irradiation therapy has been that initially inoperable cases may be rendered totally resectable by preoperative irradiation, and that a possible reduction in the number of viable cells may occur with irradiation lessening the frequency of failure.

The aforementioned considerations have made the concept of preoperative irradiation as an adjunct to surgery very attractive. However, results have in general been disappointing. Bloedorn *et al.* [2] found a one-year survival of 23% in cases treated with preoperative irradiation followed by surgical resection. Death from postoperative complications occurring as a result of irradiation was noted in 29% of patients. In a study by Bromley and Szur [3], 27% of patients developed a bronchopleural fistula or empyema following preoperative irradiation and surgery. A collaborative study under the auspices of the National Cancer Institute [9, 10] recorded no differences in survival between groups treated with preoperative irradiation and subsequent resection *versus* those treated by resection alone (and again the incidence of operative complications was increased in the preoperatively treated group). Finally, a large study by Veterans Administration [5] found preoperative irradiation to be associated with decreased survival. The complications noted in this study were not bronchopleural fistulae and empyema, but cardiovascular consequences in the postoperative period.

In summary, much of the published evidence argues against the use of preoperative irradiation as an adjunct to surgery with the single exception of superior sulcus tumors to be covered below. However, some centers continue to use this approach and have had 'favorable' results [11, 12]. Recent improvements in the results with fewer complications may very well be related to the improved delivery of irradiation by high energy equipment and better treatment planning.

2.1.2. Preoperative irradiation for superior sulcus (Pancoast) tumors. The superior sulcus tumor was first described by Pancoast in 1933 [13] as a carcinoma at the extreme apex of the lung, which often produces a typical clinical picture (shoulder pain, back pain, pain down the arm, and Horner's syndrome) due to involvement of adjacent structures such as the brachial plexus, ribs, spine, and sympathetic trunk. Paulson has advocated preoperative irradiation with 3000 rads and subsequent en bloc resection of superior sulcus pulmonary tumors together with all involved tissue [14]. As indicated in Table 2, studies by other investigators appear to support this approach when mediastinal nodes are not involved. Those studies which have reported poor results have not evaluated patients for the presence or absence of mediastinal node involvement. Although the majority of superior sulcus tumors appear to be low-grade squamous cell carcinomas, all cell

Table 2. Survival of patients with Pancoast tumor treated with preoperative irradiation and surgical resection.

Reference	Number of cases	Mediastinal involvement	5-year survival
Paulson [14]	61	no	34%
Miller *et al.* [15]	20	no	40%
Stanford *et al.* [16]	16	no	49%
Hilaris *et al.* [17]	27	no	34%
Paulson [14]	13	yes	0%
Miller *et al.* [15]	6	yes	0%

types have been represented. The need for a preoperative histological diagnosis is controversial. Many feel, as Paulson and his colleagues [18], that irradiation and operation can be undertaken on the basis of clinical diagnosis. Why preoperative irradiation is so effective in this particular circumstance is not clear, but may relate to the biology or anatomy of the tumor which provides for maximum irradiation effectiveness, good localization for adequate en bloc resection and low distant metastatic potential in relationship to other tumors within the thorax. While this combined radiotherapy-surgery approach has been recommended, other authors feel that radiotherapy alone may produce similar results [19, 20].

2.1.3. Postoperative irradiation. The rationale given for preoperative irradiation as an adjuvant to surgery applies also to postoperative irradiation with the exceptions of converting inoperable patients to operable cases. However, postoperative radiation is free from operative complications which may result from preoperative irradiation. Variable results have been reported for postoperative radiation therapy. Studies by Patterson [21] and by Gobbel [22] reported no increase in survival in operated and irradiated cases as compared to those treated with operation alone. On the other hand, Kirsh [23] has indicated that the use of postoperative irradiation in patients who are found to have tumor in mediastinal nodes at the time resection results in increased survival, particularly with squamous cell carcinomas and to a lesser extent in adenocarcinomas. A small series by Green *et al.* [24] (Table 3), supports the use of postoperative irradiation in all non-small cell cancers, regardless of histological type. Martini *et al.* [25] has

Table 3. Effect of post-operative irradiation in the treatment of non-small cell lung cancer (adapted from Green *et al.* [24].

Cell type	Positive nodes		5-year survival (surgery only/surgery + postoperative irradiation)
Squamous	none		27% / 28%
Adenocarcinoma	none		19% / 25%
Large cell anaplastic	none		9% / 25%
		Subtotal	22% / 27%
Squamous	yes		6% / 21%
Adenocarcinoma	yes		0% / 62%
Large cell anaplastic	yes		0% / 32%
		Subtotal	3% / 35%
		Total:	16% (15/94) / 31% (35/125)

recently reported the usefulness of postoperative irradiation in patients with mediastinal node involvement. Of 445 patients with mediastinal node involvement, 241 were explored, with 20% of patients surviving 3 years. Eighty cases were thought to have had complete tumor resection and of these 49% survived three years. In patients with a normal mediastinum on preoperative roentgenographic evaluation but with positive mediastinal nodes at operation, the three-year survival rate was 64%. All of these patients received postoperative irradiation. A benefit of such postoperative irradiation is sterilization of contralateral node deposits, which has been estimated to occur in approximately 6% of right-sided tumors and 27% of left-sided tumors, especially those originating in the left lower lobe [12]. No complications are associated with postoperative irradiation other than those routinely associated with thoracic irradiation. Although most physicians do not routinely employ postoperative irradiation, data now exists that would support its use. It is hoped that a large-scale trial may be undertaken to support or refute this position.

2.2. Radiation as primary treatment

In the previous section, irradiation was discussed as adjunct to surgery. In this section, irradiation is to be weighed as a primary form of treatment for non-small cell carcinoma. Most radiation oncologists believe that irradiation with intent to cure should utilize doses of at least 5000 to 6000 rads. As previously indicated, sterilization of known disease has been shown in these dose ranges [5, 26–28]. As the dose of radiation is increased, the probability for both local control and the potential for normal tissue damage increases, as demonstrated in Figure 1. The slopes may vary as well as proximity of

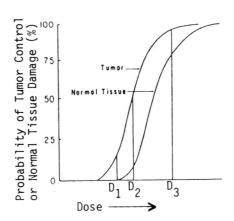

Figure 1. Probability of tumor control and normal tissue damage as a function of increase in irradiation dose. As dose increases, tumor control increases, as well as potential for normal tissue damage.

slopes depending upon individual normal tissue tolerances (i.e., skin, esophagus, spinal cord, and lung). The radiotherapist must be cognizant of these factors in determining irradiation fields and total dose. Lower doses are ineffective in terms of tumor sterilization and larger doses, as indicated above, may carry unacceptable toxicity. Several studies [26, 27] have explored the possibility that such irradiation is better administered in a split dose fashion, with delivery of roughly half of the total dose in each of two three-week periods separated by a two- or three-week rest period. Although there are several theoretical advantages to this scheme, such as the ability to reevaluate the patient prior to continuing to a higher dose, an advantage of split course over continuous irradiation has not clearly emerged.

At radiation doses of 5000–6000 rads, complications such as radiation pneumonitis, defined as an acute pneumonitis confined to radiation portals and occurring 8 to 12 weeks or sometimes longer after termination of therapy, occurs in 5 to 15% of patients; radiation fibrosis which occurs in virtually all irradiated patients to some degree usually appears 9 months or more following therapy [20]. The development of radiation fibrosis has led to the fear that curative irradiation should not be attempted in persons who cannot tolerate a pneumonectomy because of impaired pulmonary function. However, many of these patients still may be treated for cure, although their treatment portals may have to be limited to some degree. In cases where decreased pulmonary function is due to tumor obstructing blood vessels, pulmonary function is often acutely improved with radiation therapy, returning to base line or slightly below over several months depending upon the volume of lung irradiated and amount of supervening pulmonary fibrosis. Fazio *et al.* [29] have evaluated lung scans and symptoms prior to and following irradiation for lung cancer and demonstrated improvement in ventilation in 83% of patients, improvement in perfusion in 86%, and lessened breathlessness in 74% with slow deterioration of some lung function due to fibrosis over the subsequent year. These authors felt that impaired pulmonary function should not contraindicate pulmonary irradiation.

Radiation esophagitis occurs in almost all patients who receive doses above 2500 rads but usually is self-limited. More serious complications such as radiation carditis, radiation myelitis, and broncho-esophageal fistulae occur in less than 3%. One large study has recorded a radiation-related fatality rate of 2.5%, a figure somewhat higher than most other experiences. Many complications can now be avoided with modern treatment simulation and treatment planning [30, 31] and higher energy machines.

In considering radiation as a primary form of treatment in lung cancer, it must be remembered that it is a form of local treatment, in which irradiation portals encompass the primary lung lesion and potential or demonstrated regional disease. Patterns of failure must be understood to allow for

Table 4. Location of tumor causing death as a function of cell type following curative irradiation for lung cancer (from Cox *et al.* [33]).

	Local disease	Metastatic disease
Small cell	30%	70%
Adenocarcinoma	43%	57%
Large cell	45%	55%
Squamous cell	70%	30%

improvement in therapy. It is known that squamous cell carcinoma tends to metastasize less frequently than adenocarcinoma; this is an important factor in selecting therapy [32]. This point is demonstrated in an autopsy series of 300 patients who had received irradiation. As indicated in Table 4, adapted from Cox [33], most instances of squamous cell cancer deaths are associated with local progression, while most cases of small cell carcinoma die of distant spread, with adenocarcinoma deaths being intermediate with local and distant spread. Large cell undifferentiated carcinoma most closely resembled adenocarcinoma in this analysis, and other studies [34] have confirmed that it is probably most appropriate to group large cell undifferentiated cases with adenocarcinomas for purposes of planning therapy. Such data leads to the conclusion that radiation therapy would most often be curative for squamous cell carcinoma, intermediate for adenocarcinoma and large cell undifferentiated carcinoma, and infrequently curative when dealing with small cell carcinoma because of its high tendency for undetected or rapid systemic spread. Tumor doses for control are also important as shown by Sherman *et al.* [31] who showed a relationship of central control of disease to dose of radiation delivered. Central failures were noted in 50%, 22%, 18% and 5% of patients surviving more than 18 months following therapy when the amount of irradiation was 5000 rad, 5000–5500, 5500–5900, and greater than 5900 rads, respectively.

2.2.1. Irradiation of 'operable' lung cancer. In 1956 Smart and Hilton [35] described 33 cases with lung cancer considered to be candidates for operation but who were instead treated with irradiation alone. Five of these 33 patients survived for 5 years, a percentage comparable to that of a large surgical experience from that time period [8]. Although this was a retrospective, uncontrolled study, results of irradiation were surprisingly good overall and were better than the surgical series up to approximately two years following initiation of treatment. A similar study [36] comparing surgery with radiation therapy, demonstrated an advantage of surgery for long-term 'cure' although the results at one year favored irradiation. These studies indicate that surgical resection should be considered the standard form of therapy in patients with localized disease and no special surgical risk; however, if age or associated disease make resection particularly hazardous, irradiation may become the treatment of choice. In making such decisions, the risk of surgery based on age and extent of operation should be kept in mind. The surgical mortality of lobectomy in an otherwise healthy 50-year old man is 1 to 2% whereas the risk of pneumonectomy in patients over 70 may approach 40% [7]. McNeil [37] has emphasized that given the relative uncertainty of an advantage of surgery over irradiation, some elderly persons are unwilling to undergo the morbidity and mortality of surgery for uncertain long-term benefits.

2.2.2. Irradiation of 'inoperable' lung cancer. Several series have reported survival data in inoperable patients treated with radical irradiation for cure [26, 38–41]. Table 5 summarizes these results. These studies have led to some guidelines for the use of curative irradiation. Poor general condition, distant metastases, and malignant pleural effusion all contraindicate irradiation for cure; such patients are best treated for palliation when specific symptoms occur. Superior vena caval obstruction, supraclavicular metastases, and bony involvement are associated with a worse prognosis [26, 40] but are not absolute contraindications for curative irradiation. Small-sized tumors are associated with better results. If all locally inoperable lung cancer patients are irradiated for cure, Roswit [42] and Hellman [4] have demonstrated that median survival of untreated patients is only slightly prolonged with radiation therapy with a slight (4%) increase in one-year survival.

Table 5. Survival results in inoperable lung cancer treated with irradiation for cure.

Reference	Type of case	Survival (%)	
		3 years	5 years
Aristizabel and Caldwell [40]	favorable/unfavourable		16/8
Emami *et al.* [26]	favourable/unfavourable	30/11	
Coy and Kennelly [38]	age 70–90	23	17
	squamous cell		12
	other cell types		5
	(size) <3 cm/> 5 cm	26/14	
Deeley and Singh [39]		8	6
Guttman [41]		17	10

Unfavorable: superior vena caval obstruction, supraclavicular metastases, bony errosion, or undifferentiated histology.
Favorable: all others.

In the previous sections, the use of primary irradiation for curative intent has been discussed. It has also been pointed out that in many instances, patients die not only from local but also from distant metastases not appreciated at the time of initial therapy. Prophylactic brain irradiation has been used for the treatment of small cell carcinoma, to prevent distant metastasis to the brain which is a 'pharmacological sanctuary' with respect to penetration of chemotherapeutic agents. Retrospective analysis [7, 43] of the VA Lung Study Group experience suggests that prophylactic brain irradiation may be useful in non-small cell lung cancers. Brain metastases from adenocarcinomas are frequent [32] and are often found to be the single organ metastases at post-mortem examination. This data would suggest that the routine use of prophylactic brain irradiation as part of curative therapy (whether by surgery or irradiation) may be beneficial in certain patients with non-small cell lung cancer. This is another hypothesis which hopefully will be fully investigated in the future.

2.3. Palliative radiotherapy

Excellent temporary results of radiation therapy for specific complications caused by lung cancer have been noted by many authors. In patients treated for palliation only, Slawson and Scott [44] recorded control or improvement of hemoptysis in 84%, superior vena caval syndrome in 86%, arthralgias in 100%, arm and shoulder pain in 73%, chest pain in 61%, and dyspnea in 60%. Results were less impressive in treatment of atelectasis (23% improvement) or vocal cord paralysis (6% improvement). Dyspnea may often be temporarily improved by radiation. Cases in which dyspnea is most likely to be benefited by irradiation may be detected by lung scanning, which usually reveals larger perfusion and ventilation defect than would be anticipated from the chest X-ray, presumably due to the effect of mediastinal metastases on pulmonary vessels and bronchi. Many authors have demonstrated the effectiveness of 'spot' radiation for local bone symptoms in metastatic lung cancer, as well as from metastatic disease of other malignancies [45]. However, many patients experience multiple areas of metastasis. In recent years, hemi-body radiotherapy has shown promise in relief of symptoms in such situations [45, 46].

2.4. New advances in radiation therapy

With the recent development of computerized axial tomography, tumor volume can be more accurately defined. This may lead to smaller radiation portals, better definition of tumor and normal tissues which may allow for higher tumor volume doses and minimal increases in normal tissue complications. The use of radiation sensitizers or radiation protectors is now being investigated in the laboratoy and in a few clinical trials; such sensitizers may lead to a gain in the therapeutic ratio. Brachytherapy is not new, however, it has not been used routinely; Hilaris and his colleagues have demonstrated its benefit [47]. Recent publication by Abe and his co-workers [48] in Japan and preliminary studies in the United States suggest that intraoperative irradiation of the tumor bed may be effective in giving high tumor doses of radiation with limited normal tissue irradiation. The possibility that postoperative irradiation might be found to be applicable to most cases has been mentioned previously, as has the possibility of prophylactic cranial irradiation in adenocarcinoma. Investigations into the use of tightly targeted irradiation excluding the mediastinum for patients with small peripheral lesions and who are pulmonary cripples are needed. It is possible that such treatment may be associated with only minimal loss of pulmonary function since it is the inclusion of the mediastinum in the irradiated field which extends the volume of pulmonary parenchyma subjected to irradiation. It is well known that a large number of patients who fail primary treatment relapse in the primary site or with distant metastases in non-small cell carcinoma. In recent years, trials of chemotherapy combined with radiotherapy have emerged as discussed in subsequent sections. The difficulty at this time is determining effective chemotherapy agents, sequence of combination therapy, and the morbidity of the combined treatments. More studies are needed to answer these questions and the effectiveness of this type of combined therapy.

2.5. Summary and conclusions regarding radiation therapy of non-small cell lung cancer

The following conclusions and recommendations seem reasonable at the present time from these data discussed above: (1) curative radiation for patients with localized but inoperable non-small cell lung carcinoma is appropriate for those who are in relatively good physical condition. Bony invasion or superior vena caval obstruction will compromise results, but are not absolute contraindications; (2) for clinically operable patients in whom advanced age or associated medical illness causes an increased operative risk, irradiation therapy may be an acceptable alternative treatment; (3) preoperative irradiation in most studies has not demonstrated an increase in survival although further controlled studies may be needed to clarify its efficacy. An exception are the superior sulcus tumors without mediastinal involvement in which preoperative irradiation and resection of involved tissues provides a 30 to 50% five-year survival; (4) postoperative irradiation appears to be indicated in patients with mediastinal nodes removed at operation particularly for patients with squamous cell histology; (5) palliative irradiation for symptoms is often helpful; (6) cranial prophylactic irradiation may be indicated in adenocarcinoma of the lung regardless of treatment modality; (7) new diagnostic techniques and improved treatment planning may allow increase in doses with concomitant increase in local control; (8) higher local doses may be given with the use of interstitial brachytherapy or intraoperative treatment.

3. CHEMOTHERAPY OF NON-SMALL CELL CARCINOMA OF THE LUNG

Antineoplastic chemotherapy, in contrast to surgery or radiation therapy, is a systemic form of therapy and has an advantage over other forms of cancer treatment in its potential ability to kill malignant cells throughout the body. As nearly as 50% of patients with lung cancer have distant metastasis at the time of diagnosis and another 40% develop locally recurrent or distal spread of their disease following initial treatment with surgery or radiation therapy [49], the advantage of a systemic form of effective therapy for non-small cell lung cancer is of major potential benefit. Of the nearly 125,000 patients in the United States diagnosed as having lung cancer in 1982, 112,000 or 90% will initially or eventually be candidates for systemic chemotherapy if such treatment could be shown to be of significant therapeutic usefulness. Unfortunately unlike small cell carcinoma of the lung, clinical trials using chemotherapy for treatment of non-small cell lung cancer have not consistently demonstrated a clinical benefit to patients with this disease, although recent studies have indicated some progress in the development of drug combinations which may help specific groups of patients with non-small cell lung cancer. Care must be taken by clinicians reviewing results of studies of chemotherapeutic trials of non-small cell lung cancer to be cognizant of factors other than drug treatment which are important in determining response rates and survival of patients with non-small cell lung cancer and may bias conclusions made in such studies.

3.1. Factors influencing response rates and survival of patients with non-small cell lung cancer

Reviewing published studies of chemotherapeutic trials in non-small cell lung cancer may confuse many physicians. Tumor shrinkage has been reported to occur in 5–57% of patients treated with various chemotherapeutic regimens [50, 51] and the reported median survival of patients treated with chemotherapy has varied from 2.5–9.0 months [52, 53]. This wide variation in treatment results is related in some degree to the type of therapy used, but also represents selection of different groups of patients with varying prognostic factors. The two most common methods for analyzing the results of treatment for non-small cell lung cancer have been comparison of the survival of treated with nontreated patients (often histo-

Table 6. Karnofsky performance status.

%	Criteria
100	Normal; no complaints; no evidence of disease.
90	Able to carry on normal activity; minor signs or symptoms of disease.
80	Normal activity with effort; some signs or symptoms of disease.
70	Cares for self; unable to carry on normal activity or to do active work.
60	Requires occasional assistance, but is able to care for most of his needs.
50	Requires considerable assistance and frequent medical care.
40	Disabled; require special care and assistance.
30	Severely disabled; hospitalization is indicated although death not imminent.
20	Very sick; hospitalization necessary; active supportive treatment necessary.
10	Moribund; fatal processes progressing rapidly.
0	Dead.

rical controls) and the number of patients having a response (shrinkage of tumor) with treatment. Several studies have recently indicated that both survival duration and response rates are dependent upon the patient's initial performance status, spread of disease, and degree of weight loss at the time of diagnosis. Stanley [54] has analyzed the survival results of over 5000 patients with inoperable bronchogenic carcinoma of the lung followed by the Veterans Administration Lung Group in terms of 77 potential prognostic factors. Performance status, extent of disease, and degree of weight loss in the 6 months prior to diagnosis were found to be the most important prognostic factors for survival with initial performance status being the dominant prognostic factor. The effect of Karnofsky performance status (Table 6), the effect of disease spread, and the degree of weight loss on median survival are shown in Table 7. Using these 3 prognostic variables, median survival of patients with inoperable non-small cell lung cancer can vary from 6 weeks to more than 1 year. Such factors must be recognized when evaluating trials of chemotherapy on the basis of median survival.

The second major assessment for evaluating the benefits of chemotherapy in the treatment of non-small cell lung cancer is the quantitation of the number of patients whose tumor shrinks with drug treatment. Responses to chemotherapy have been generally assessed by standard response criteria, i.e. a complete response is defined as disappearance of all disease for at least one month and a partial response defined as a 50% decrease in the products of the greatest perpendicular diameters of one or more measurable lesions which lasts one month and is not accompanied by increasing lesions elsewhere. Recently, Eagan [55] has enlarged the definition for response to include a definite decrease in tumor size agreed upon by two investigators

Table 7. Median survival estimates (in weeks).

Initial performance status	Disease confined to one hemithorax			Disease extending beyond one hemithorax					
				No scalene or supraclavicular nodal involvement			Scalene and/or supraclavicular nodal involvement		
	No weight loss	Weight loss <10%	Weight loss >10%	No weight loss	Weight loss <10%	Weight loss >10%	No weight loss	Weight loss <10%	Weight loss >10%
100	72	54	43	41	31	26	33	26	21
90	55	41	33	32	25	20	26	20	17
80	48	36	30	29	22	18	23	18	15
70	42	32	27	26	20	16	21	16	13
60	33	26	21	20	16	13	16	13	10
50	26	20	17	16	12	10	13	10	8
40	21	16	13	10	8	10	10	7	6

From Stanley [54] with approval of the author and the Journal of the National Cancer Institute.

Table 8. Response rate to chemotherapy in non-small cell lung cancer as a function of patient performance status.

	Published response rates in various series					
	Bedikian *et al.* [55]	Bitran *et al.* [56]	Lad *et al.* [57]	Richards *et al.* [58]	Vincent *et al.* [59]	Chahinian *et al.* [60]
Fully ambulatory	25%	52%	23%	55%	21%	64%
Bedrideen 5–50% of day	14%	30%	–	–	–	50%
Confined to bed over 50% of day	–	0%	8%	5%	9%	41%

with no new lesions appearing. This criteria allows assessment of tumor response in those patients in whom tumor diameters are not easily measured due to tumor abutting normal intrathoracic structures. Using these criteria, the Mayo Clinic group has been unable to detect differences in regression rates, time to regression, duration of response or survival between patients followed by 'measurable' or by 'evaluable' criteria and have suggested that 'evaluable criteria' should be used in future studies. The type of response criteria used for evaluating results of chemotherapeutic trials must be carefully noted by each reader.

Performance status and extent of disease spread have been shown to predict not only for survival but also for response of a patient's disease to treatment with antineoplastic drugs. No matter what criteria are used, responses to chemotherapy are usually seen in those patients with the best performance status. In several series (Table 8), highest response rates have been seen in those patients who are fully ambulatory while patients who are confined to bed more than 50% of the day have little chance of responding to chemotherapeutic treatment. Evaluation of response rates to various chemotherapeutic regimens needs to be considered in light of patients performance status before entry into study.

Histologic subclassification and effect of prior irradiation therapy may also be important prognostic factors in evaluating survival and response rates in non-small cell lung cancer. However, to date, there is insufficient data on either of these two prognostic factors to assess their impact on results of chemotherapeutic trials [61, 62]. As treatment improves it is possible that the importance of such factors will be identified.

3.2. Single agent chemotherapy

A number of individual drugs have been reported to produce tumor

Table 9. Single agent chemotherapy in non-small cell lung cancer.

Drug	Response rate
Vindesine	20%
Mitomycin-C	20%
VP-16	15%
Doxorubicin	15%
Cisplatin	15%
Cyclophosphamide	10%

Response rates estimated by authors from averages of data reported in [63–75].

shrinkage in a small proportion of patients with non-small cell lung cancer. Exact response rates for individual drugs are difficult to determine due to a wide variation in reported response rates. As an example, response rates of 4–51% have been reported for cyclophosphamide when used as a single agent [50, 63, 64]. These variations may be the result of different patient selection (performance status, extent of disease, previous chemotherapy, etc.), drug doses, or response criteria. Table 9 indicates approximate response rates for single agents showing greatest activity against non-small cell lung cancer. As can be noted, activity of single agents is considerably less than that seen in treatment of small cell lung cancer and further development of new drugs for non-small cell lung cancer is needed. Responses to single agent chemotherapy, when achieved, are usually of short duration (2–4 months) and no prolongation in survival for patients treated with single agent chemotherapy has been noted in most studies including a large randomized study conducted by the Veterans Administration Lung Cancer Study Group looking at treatment with nitrogen mustard and cyclophosphamide [70].

3.3. Combination chemotherapy

The combined use of several antineoplastic agents with nonoverlapping toxicity has been more effective in producing higher response rates, longer survival and a greater chance for cure than therapy with single drugs in the treatment of most sensitive malignancies [76]. Such results have led to a host of clinical trials of combination chemotherapy for the treatment of inoperable non-small cell lung cancer despite the lack of available drugs with more than a 25% response rate when used as single agents. Most trials of combination chemotherapy have not been randomized but have been compared with historical controls. Therefore, results need to be carefully analyzed with particular attention to prognostic factors outlined earlier. The majority of published trials have reported response rates of less than 40%

Table 10. Chemotherapy regimens showing response rates of more than forty percent in non-small cell lung cancer.

Drug regimen	Number of patients	Total response rate	Complete response rate	Median survival (months)	Reference
CM	41	49%	7%	8.0	Straus [77, 78]
T-CAP	35	57%	3%	7.3	Eagan *et al.* [51]
CAP	42	48%	0%	5.8	Eagan *et al.* [79]
MOCPr	28	43%	0%	NS	Alberts *et al.* [80]
BACON	50	42%	4%	5.0	Livingston *et al.* [81]
FOMi	52	41%	7%	6.0	Miller *et al.* [82]
VP (low dose)	55	46%	7%	NS	Gralla *et al.* [83]
VP (high dose)	52	40%	13%	NS	Gralla *et al.* [83]
MACCx	68	44%	4%	8.3	Chahinian *et al.* [60]
CAMPr	37	44%	3%	6.4	Lad *et al.* [84]

C = cyclophosphamide; T = traizinate; A = doxorubicin (Adriamycin®); P = cisplatin; M = methotrexate; O = vincristine (Oncouin®); Pr = procarbazine; N = nitrogen mustard; Mi = mitomycin-C; Cx = lomustine (CCNU); NS = not stated.

with median survival of all treated patients of 3–6 months. A few studies (Table 10) have been reported which do show response rates of over 40% and a few of these have a median survival of greater than 8 months. When these results are compared to the natural history of untreated, inoperable (both limited and extensive disease) lung cancer which has a median survival of 5–6 months for ambulatory patients and 2–3 months for nonambulatory patients [70, 85], these treatment regimens appear to offer some benefit in the therapy of this disease. Unfortunately, treatment results with some of these combinations, such as vindesine and cisplatin, have not yet been confirmed and repeat investigations of many drug combinations have not been able to duplicate initially encouraging studies (Table 11). With the wide variation in response rates and the modest prolongation in survival noted in reported studies, no presently available combination chemotherapy regimen can be recommended as standard therapy for inoperable non-small cell lung cancer. Patients responding to chemotherapy do appear to benefit from such treatment. In nearly all reported studies, there is a significant prolongation in life for patients responding to chemotherapy when compared to those patients not responding (Table 12). However, as previously mentioned, patients with better initial performance status are more likely to respond to chemotherapy and this is also the group of patients with the longest median survival when untreated. Thus, as pointed out by Aisner and Hansen [99], there is presently no clear-cut evidence that any combination

Table 11. Results of repeated clinical trials of certain combination chemotherapy regimens in the treatment of non-small cell lung cancer.

Drug combination	Response rate	Median survival	Year reported	Reference
CM	49%	8.0 months	1979	Straus [77, 78]
CM	13%	6.0 months	1981	Creech *et al.* [86]
BACON	42%	5.0 months	1976	Livingston *et al.* [81]
BACON	21%	4.0 months	1977	Livingston *et al.* [87]
MACC	38%	6.6 months	1977	Chahinian *et al.* [88]
MACC	44%	8.3 months	1979	Chahinian *et al.* [60]
MACC	12%	3.8 months	1979	Vogl *et al.* [89]
MACC	12%	3.5 months	1981	Ruckdeschel *et al.* [90]
CAMP	27%	5.1 months	1978	Bitran *et al.* [91]
CAMP	31%	N.S.	1979	Lad *et al.* [57]
CAMP	17%	6.0 months	1981	Cambareri *et al.* [92]
CAMP	22%	5.0 months	1981	Ruckdeschel *et al.* [93]
CAMP	44%	6.4 months	1981	Lad *et al.* [84]
CAP	42%	6.8 months	1978	Britell *et al.* [66]
CAP	48%	5.8 months	1979	Eagan *et al.* [51]
CAP	28%	6.0 months	1979	Gralla *et al.* [69]
CAP	29%	3.9 months	1981	Evans *et al.* [94]
CAP	35%	7.6 months	1981	Knost *et al.* [95]
CAP	8%	3.3 months	1981	Robert *et al.* [96]
CAP	7%	5.4 months	1981	Davis *et al.* [97]

Table 12. Effect of response to chemotherapy on survival in non-small cell carcinoma of the lung.

Median survival of responders	Median survival of non-responders	p value	Reference
6.5	2.2	0.002	Livingston *et al.* [81]
9.9	2.8	0.001	Livingston *et al.* [87]
12.6	2.4	0.001	Bitran *et al.* [91]
12.3	4.7	0.001	Lad *et al.* [57]
9.0	3.0	0.001	Langotte *et al.* [98]
21.7	6.0	0.01	Gralla *et al.* [83]
12.6	4.3	NS	Knost *et al.* [95]
8.3	2.4	0.001	Evans *et al.* [94]
8.0	4.5	0.02	Ruckdeschel *et al.* [90]
8.0	4.0	0.002	Ruckdeschel *et al.* 893]
12.0	4.3	0.005	Chahinian *et al.* [60]

chemotherapy regimen is superior to no treatment or produces such an effect independent of predetermined prognostic factors.

A few as of yet unconfirmed studies suggest recent improvement in the chemotherapeutic treatment of non-small cell lung cancer. Combinations containing mitomycin-C appear to be active [74, 82]. Gralla *et al.* [83] have presented data on the use of vindesine and cisplatin which is encouraging and should lead to further studies investigating this combination. These authors randomized 85 patients (82 with distant metastasis) with squamous cell and adenocarcinoma of the lung to therapy with 3 mg/m^2 vindesine and either high-dose (120 mg/m^2) or low-dose 60 mg/m^2) cisplatin. Both treatment regimens produced remission rates of 40–45%. However, the duration of remission (12 *vs* 5.5 months) and the median survival of responding patients (21.7 *vs* 10 months) was significantly greater for patients being treated with high-dose cisplatin. The 12-month remission duration is significantly greater than remission durations reported with other chemotherapeutic combinations. Confirmatory studies are needed before this treatment can be recommended for routine medical practice.

The toxicity of combination chemotherapeutic regimens used for the treatment of non-small cell lung cancer is significant. The Eastern Cooperative Oncology Group has noted an overall incidence of severe toxicity of 19%, life-threatening toxicity of 9%, and a 3% incidence of drug-related deaths resulting from different chemotherapeutic regimens used for the therapy of non-small cell lung cancer from 1975–1980 [100]. Toxicities vary to some extent with the specific chemotherapeutic regimen used. Nausea and vomiting are common with most drug combinations and may be severe; in a study by Vogelzang [101], 16% of patients declined further chemotherapy because of gastrointestinal side effects. Myelosuppression is also frequent and the most common cause of mortality and morbidity. Other toxicities, such as nephropathy due to cisplatin or neuropathy from vincristine or vindesine, are noted at differing frequencies depending upon the specific treatment program. Table 13 lists toxicity frequencies associated with some of the more commonly used regimens for the treatment of non-small cell lung cancer.

3.4. Recommendations for use of combination chemotherapy in the treatment of non-small cell carcinoma of the lung

Since presently available chemotherapeutic regimens are only rarely (case reports [103, 104]) associated with long-term disease-free survival, produce only minimal prolongation of median survival, and have significant toxicity, no combination chemotherapeutic regimen can be recommended as standard therapy for patients with disseminated non-small cell lung cancer. We would currently recommend that patients with this disease who desire

209

Table 13. Toxicity of selected chemotherapeutic regimens used for treatment of non-small cell lung cancer.

Drug combination	Reference	Incidence of nausea and vomiting	Mean WBC or granulocyte nadir	Mean platelet nadir	Incidence of nephrotoxicity	Incidence of neuropathy	Incidence of alopecia	Incidence of drug-related mortality
CAP	[80]	100%	2600/mm³ (WBC)	90,000/mm³	19%	–	100%	0%
COMB	[102]	NS	600/mm³ (polys)	140,000/mm³	–	11%	17%	6%
MACCx	[60]	100%	1600/mm³ (WBC)	63,000/mm³	5%	–	100%	1%
BACON	[87]	100%	1100/mm³ (polys)	145,000/mm³	–	–	100%	4%
CAMPr	[91]	100%	1200/mm³ (polys)	135,000/mm³	–	–	100%	4%
V-P	[83]	100%	2700/mm³ (WBC)	195,000/mm³	38%	100%	66%	0%

therapy be referred to oncology centers investigating new treatments of non-small cell lung cancer. If such a referral cannot be made, treatment with a combination such as cyclophosphamide, adriamycin, cisplatin (CAP) or vindesine-cisplatin may be tried in certain patients desiring therapy. These patients need to understand and accept the limited benefits presently available and be able to tolerate expected toxicities. Only patients with Karnofsky performance status of 70 or better, no prior chemotherapy treatment, and those having measurable disease should be considered for chemotherapy. Treatment should follow published protocols carefully and must be administered by a physician who has experience in giving such drugs and has facilities to support patients should complications arise. If no evidence of tumor shrinkage is noted following 2 cycles of therapy, treatment should be discontinued to avoid further toxicity to the patient. In those patients in whom a response to treatment is noted, additional courses may be employed until disease progression is noted or for a 1–2-year period in those few patients achieving a complete remission.

3.5. Combined surgery and chemotherapy

Tumor recurrence following potentially curative surgery remains a major medical problem, particularly in patients with pathologic Stage II and III disease. A number of studies using chemotherapy as an adjuvant to potentially curative surgery in hopes of improving the overall cure rate have been undertaken during the past decade. Administration of chemotherapy at a time when tumor cell burden is low and the tumor growth fraction is high is theoretically attractive and use of adjuvant chemotherapy in such a setting has been of clinical benefit in the treatment of Wilm's tumors, breast cancer, and osteogenic sarcoma. Unfortunately, no studies to date have indicated that adjuvant chemotherapy improves median survival or 5-year cure rate over surgery alone in the treatment of non-small cell lung cancer. The Veterans Administration Surgical Adjuvant Group has investigated the use of nitrogen mustard, cyclophosphamide, and methotrexate as an adjuvant to surgery alone [105–107]. Of a total of 2,348 curative resections, 1,176 patients received only surgery while 1,172 were randomized to receive adjuvant chemotherapy. Five- and 10-year survival rates for treated patients were 24.8% and 13.5%; control patients treated with surgery alone had 5- and 10-year survivals of 26.2 and 16.3%. No specific drug was found to be effective. The combinations of cyclophosphamide plus methotrexate and CCNU plus hydroxyurea have also been found to be ineffective in similar studies by the same group. Controlled studies by the British Medical Research Council have also shown a lack of benefit of single agent chemotherapy as an adjuvant to surgery [108]. Although uncontrolled trials have been published suggesting improved survival using adjuvant chemotherapy, most studies to date do not support such a view [109] and we feel there is no good evidence to recommend the use of adjuvant chemotherapy except in an investigative setting. As more effective chemotherapy for disseminated non-small cell lung cancer is developed, use of such effective combinations in an adjuvant setting may prove beneficial. The Lung Cancer Study Group is currently investigating the use of cyclophosphamide, adriamycin, and cisplatin (CAP) in an adjuvant setting.

3.6. Combined use of radiation therapy and chemotherapy

Antineoplastic chemotherapy has been combined with radiation therapy in an attempt to improve the median survival and cure rate over that achieved with radiation therapy alone. Randomized controlled trials using cyclophosphamide, 5-fluorouracil, nitrogen mustard and other single agents have not shown any clinical benefit over results achieved with radiation therapy alone [110–112]. Although conclusions from published reports vary from a slight advantage to the addition of chemotherapy [113] to a slight increase in toxicity with no therapeutic benefit [110], the bulk of data indicates that single agent chemotherapy does not change the survival of lung cancer patients treated with radiation therapy alone. Similar results have also been found when combination chemotherapy consisting of CCNU plus methotrexate plus cyclophosphamide is added to high-dose (4000 rad) radiation therapy [110].

Occasional uncontrolled trials have reported results of combined surgery, radiation therapy, and chemotherapy for localized inoperable cancer. Takita et al. [114] have treated 24 selected patients with localized inoperable non-small cell lung cancer with various cisplatin containing combination chemotherapy regimens followed by surgical resection, irradiation, and more chemotherapy. Median survival of this group of patients from initiation of therapy was 11 months with 3 patients alive at over 2 years following treatment. It appears that occasionally long-term survivors are seen following aggressive multimodality treatment programs such as this but unfortunately none of the studies have been controlled and similar results may potentially be found with radiation therapy alone. Therefore, treatment programs employing the combined use of surgery, radiation therapy and chemotherapy in any sequence must, for the time being, be considered investigational.

REFERENCES

1. Silverberg E: Cancer Statistics, 1982. CA – A Journal for Clinicians 32:15–32, 1982.
2. Bloedorn FG, Cowley RA, Cuccia CA, et al.: Preoperative irradiation in bronchogenic carcinoma. Am J Roent 92:77–87, 1964.
3. Bromley LL, Szur L: Combined radiotherapy and resection for carcinoma of the bronchus. Lancet 2:937–941, 1955.

212

4. Hellman S, Kligerman M, Von Essen C, *et al.*: Sequelae of radical radiotherapy of carcinoma of the lung. Radiology 182: 1055–1061, 1964.
5. Shields TW: Preoperative radiation therapy in the treatment of bronchial carcinoma. Cancer 30: 1388–1394, 1972.
6. Rissanen PM, Tikka U, Holsti LR: Autopsy findings in lung cancer treated with megavoltage radiotherapy. Acta Radiologica 7:433–442, 1968.
7. Higgins GA, Beebe GW: Bronchogenic carcinoma; Factors in survival. Arch Surg 94: 539–549, 1967.
8. Bignall JR, Moon AJ: Survival after lung resection for bronchial carcinoma. Thorax 10:183-190, 1955.
9. Collaborative Study: Preoperative irradiation of cancer of the lung: Preliminary report of a therapeutic trial. Cancer 23:419–430, 1969.
10. Collaborative Study: Preoperative irradiation of cancer of the lung. Final report of a therapeutic trial. Cancer 36:914–925, 1975.
11. Sherman DM, Neptune W, Weichelsbaum RR, *et al.*: An aggressive approach to marginally resectable lung cancer. Cancer 41:204–205, 1978.
12. Kirschner PA: Lung cancer – surgical significance of mediastinal lymph node metastases. NY State J Med 79:2036–2041, 1979.
13. Pancoast HK: Superior pulmonary sulcus tumor: Tumor characterized by pain, Horner's syndrome, destruction of bone and atrophy of hand muscles. JAMA 99:1391–1396, 1932.
14. Paulson DL: Carcinomas in the superior pulmonary sulcus. J Thoracic Cardiovasc Surg 70:1095-1104, 1975.
15. Miller J, Mansour K, Hatcher C: Carcinoma of the superior pulmonary sulcus. Ann Thoracic |Surg 28:44–47, 1979.
16. Stanford W, Barnes R, Tucker T: Influences of staging in superior sulcus (Pancoast) tumors of the lung. Ann Thoracic Surg 29:406–409, 1980.
17. Hilaris B, Luomanen R, Beattie E: Integrated irradiation and surgery in the treatment of apical lung cancer. Cancer 27:1369–1373, 1971.
18. Mallams JT, Paulson DL, Collier RE, *et al.*: Presurgical irradiation in bronchogenic carcinoma, superior sulcus type. Radiology 82:1050–1054, 1964.
19. Komaki R, Roh J, Cox JD, *et al.*: Superior sulcus tumors: Results of irradiation of 36 patients. Cancer 48:1563–1568, 1981.
20. Libshitz H. Southard M: Complications of radiation therapy: Seminars Roent 9:41–49, 1974.
21. Patterson R and Russell MH: Clinical trials in malignant disease. Part IV – Lung Cancer. Value of postoperative radiotherapy. Clin Radiol 13:141–144, 1962.
22. Gobbel WG, Sawyers JL, Rhea WG: Experience with palliative resection and irradiation therapy for carcinoma of the lung. J Thoracic Cardiovasc Surg 53:183–191, 1967.
23. Kirsh M, Rotman H, Argenta L, *et al.*: Carcinoma of the lung: Results of treatment over ten years. Ann Thoracic Surg 21:371–377, 1976.
24. Green N, Kurohara SS, George FW III, *et al.*: Post resection irradiation for primary lung cancer. Radiology 116:405–407, 1975.
25. Martini N, Flehninger B, Zaman M, *et al.*: Prospective study of 445 lung carcinomas with mediastinal lymph node metastases. J Thoracic Cardiovasc Surg 80:390–399, 1980.
26. Emami B, Munzenrider J, Lee D, *et al.*: Radical radiation therapy of advanced lung cancer. Evaluation of prognostic factors and results of continuous and split course treatment. Cancer 44:446–456, 1979.
27. Perez CA, Stanley K, Rubin P, *et al.*: A prospective randomized study of various irradiation doses and fractionation schedule in the treatment of inoperable non-oat cell carcinoma of the lung. Cancer 45:2744–2753, 1980.

28. Petrovich Z, Mietlowski W, Ohanian M, *et al.*: Clinical report on the treatment of locally advanced lung cancer. Cancer 40:72–77, 1977.

29. Fazio F, Pratt T, McKenzie C, *et al.*: Improvement in regional ventilation and perfusion after radiotherapy for unresectable carcinoma of the bronchus. Am J Roent 133:191–200, 1979.

30. Dritschilo A, Sherman D, Emami B, *et al.*: The cost effectiveness of radiation therapy simulator: a model for the determination of need. Int J Rad Onc Bio Phys 5:243–247, 1979.

31. Sherman DM, Weichelsbaum RR, Hellman S: The characteristics of long-term survivors of lung cancer treated with radiation. Cancer 47:2575–2580, 1981.

32. Matthews M, Kanhouwa S, Pickeren J, *et al.*: Frequency of residual and metastatic tumor in patients undergoing curative surgical resection for lung cancer. Cancer Chemotherapy Rep 4:63–67, 1973.

33. Cox J, Yesner R, Mietlowski W, *et al.*: Influence of cell type on failure pattern after irradiation for locally advanced carcinoma of the lung. Cancer 44:94–98, 1979.

34. Mitchell D, Morgan P, Ball J: Prognostic features of large cell anaplastic carcinoma of the bronchus. Thorax 35:118–122, 1980.

35. Smart J, Hilton G: Radiotherapy·of cancer of the lung. Results in a selected group of cases. Lancet 1:880–881, 1956.

36. Morrison R, Deeley TJ, Cleland WP: The treatment of carcinoma of the bronchus. A clinical trial to compare surgery and supravoltage radiotherapy. Lancet 1:683–684, 1963.

37. McNeil B, Weichselbaum R, Pauker S: Fallacy of the five-year survival in lung cancer. N Engl J Med 292:1397–1401, 1978.

38. Coy P, Kennelly GM: The role of curative radiotherapy in the treatment of lung cancer. Cancer 45:698–702, 1980.

39. Deeley TJ, Singh SP: Treatment of inoperable carcinoma of the bronchus by megavoltage X-rays. Thorax 22:562–566, 1967.

40. Aristizabel SA, Caldwell WL: Radical irradiation with the split course technique in carcinoma of the lung. Cancer 37:2630–2635, 1976.

41. Guttman RJ: Effectiveness of radiotherapy in explored inoperable carcinoma of the lung. Bull NY Acad Med 45:657–664, 1969.

42. Roswit B, Patmo ME, Rapp R, *et al.*: The survival of patients with inoperable lung cancer: a large-scale randomized study of radiation therapy *versus* placebo. Radiology 90:688–697, 1968.

43. Cox J, Yesner R: Adenocarcinoma of the lung: Recent results from the Veterans Administration Lung Group. Am Rev Resp Dis 120:1025–1029, 1979.

44. Slawson R, Scott R: Radiation therapy for bronchogenic carcinoma. Radiology 132:175–176, 1979.

45. Hendrickson FR, Shehata WM, Kirchner AB: Radiation therapy for osseous metastasis. Int J Rad Onc Bio Phys 1:275–278, 1976.

46. Fitzpatrick PJ, Rider WD: Half body radiotherapy. Int J Rad Onc Bio Phys 1:197–207, 1976.

47. Hilaris B, Martini M: Interstitial brachytherapy in cancer of the lung: a 20-year experience. Int J Rad Onc Biol Phys 5:1951–1956, 1979.

48. Abe M, Takahashi M, Yabumoto E, *et al.*: Clinical experiences with intraoperative radiotherapy of locally advanced cancers. Cancer 45:40–48, 1980.

49. Benfield JR, Juillard GJ, Pilch YH, *et al.*: Current and future concepts of lung cancer. Ann Intern Med 83:93–106, 1975.

50. Bodey G, Lagakos S, Gutierrez A, *et al.*: Therapy of advanced squamous cell carcinoma of the lung: Cyclophosphamide *vs* COMB. Cancer 39:1026–1031, 1977.

51. Eagan RT, Frytak S, Ingle J, *et al.*: Phase II evaluation of the combination of triazinate, cyclophosphamide, doxorubicin and cis-diamminedichloroplatinum in patients with advanced adenocarcinoma of the lung. Cancer Treat Rep 64:925–928, 1980.

52. Ihde DC, Cohen MH, Bunn PA, *et al.*: Bleomycin, methotrexate and streptozotocin in epidermoid carcinoma of the lung. An active drug combination with major non-hematologic toxicity. Cancer Treat Rep 62:155–157, 1978.

53. Bedikian A, Staab R, Livingston R, *et al.*: Chemotherapy for adenocarcinoma of the lung with 5-fluorouracil, cyclophosphamide, and CCNU. Cancer 44:858–863, 1979.

54. Stanley KE: Prognostic factors for survival in patients with inoperable lung cancer. JNCI 65:25–32, 1980.

55. Eagan RT, Fleming TR, Schoonover V: Evaluation of response criteria in advanced lung cancer. Cancer 44:1125–1128, 1979.

56. Bitran JD, Desser RK, DeMeester T, *et al.*: Combined modality therapy for stage III$_{Mo}$ non-oat cell bronchogenic carcinoma. Cancer Treat Rep. 62:327–332, 1978.

57. Lad T, Sarma R, Diekamp U, *et al.*: 'CAMP' combination chemotherapy for unresectable non-oat cell bronchogenic carcinoma. Cancer Clinical Trials 2:321–326, 1979.

58. Richards F, White D, Muss H, *et al.*: Combination chemotherapy of advanced non-oat cell carcinoma of the lung. Cancer 44:1576–1581, 1979.

59. Vincent R, Mehta C, Tucker R, *et al.*: Chemotherapy of extensive large cell and adenocarcinoma of the lung. Cancer 46:256–260, 1980.

60. Chahinian A, Mandel EM, Holland JF, *et al.*: MACC (methotrexate, adriamycin, cyclophosphamide and CCNU) in advanced lung cancer. Cancer 43:1590–1597, 1979.

61. Livingston RB, Heilbrun LH: Patterns of response and relapse in chemotherapy of extensive squamous carcinoma of the lung. Cancer Chemo Pharmacol 1:225–227, 1980.

62. Hande KR, Des Prez RM: Chemotherapy and radiation therapy of non-small cell lung carcinoma. Clin Chest Med 3:399–414, 1982.

63. Barron KM, Helm WH, King DA: Bronchial carcinoma treated with nitrogen mustard and cyclophosphamide. Br Med J 2:685–687, 1965.

64. Cohen M, Perevodchikova N: Single agent chemotherapy of lung cancer. In: Progress in Cancer Research and Therapy. Muggia FM, Rosenzweig M (eds). New York, NY: Raven Press, Vol 11, 1979, p 343.

65. Rossof AH, Bearden JD, Coltman CA: Phase II evaluation of cis-diamminedichloroplatinum (II) in lung cancer. Cancer Treat Rep 60:1679–1686, 1976.

66. Britell JC, Eagan RT, Ingle JN, *et al.*: Cis-dichlorodiammineplatinum alone followed by adriamycin plus cyclophosphamide at progression *vs* cis-dichlorodiammineplatinum, adriamycin and cyclophosphamide in combination for adenocarcinoma of the lung. Cancer Treat Rep 62: 1207–1210, 1978.

67. Natale RB, Gralla RJ, Wittes RE, *et al.*: Vindesine chemotherapy in lung cancer. Cancer Treat Reviews 7:59–63, 1980.

68. DeJager R, Longeval E, Klastersky J: High-dose cisplatin with fluid and manitol induced diuresis in advanced lung cancer. A Phase II clinical trial of the EORTC Lung Cancer Working Party. Cancer Treat Rep 64: 1341–1346, 1980.

69. Gralla RJ, Cvitkovic E, Golbey RB: Cis-dichlorodiammineplatinum in non-small cell lung carcinoma of the lung. Cancer Treat Rep 63:1585–1588, 1979.

70. Green RA, Humphrey E, Close H, *et al.*: Alkylating agents in bronchogenic carcinoma. Am. J Med 46:516–525, 1969.

71. Livingston RB: Combination chemotherapy of bronchogenic carcinoma: non-oat cell. Cancer Treat Reviews 4:153–165, 1977.

72. Selawry O: Chemotherapy in lung cancer. In: Lung Cancer: Clinical Diagnosis and Treatment. Straus MJ (ed). New York, NY: Grune and Stratton, 1977, p 199.

73. Blum RH: An overview of studies with adriamycin (NSC-123127) in the United States. Cancer Chemotherapy Rep 6:247–251, 1975.

74. Samson MJ, Comis RL, Baker LH, *et al.*: Mitomycin-C in advanced adenocarcinoma and large cell carcinoma of the lung. Cancer Treat Rep 62: 163–165, 1978.

75. Eagan RT, Ingle JN, Creagan ET, *et al.*: VP-16 chemotherapy for advanced adenocarcinoma and large cell carcinoma of the lung. Cancer Treat Rep 62:843–844, 1978.

76. DeVita VT, Schein PS: The use of drugs in combination for the treatment of cancer. N Engl J Med 288:998–1006, 1973.

77. Straus MJ: Cytokinetic chemotherapy design for the treatment of advanced lung cancer. Cancer Treat Rep 63:767–773, 1979.

78. Straus MJ: Combination chemotherapy in advanced lung cancer with increased survival. Cancer 38:2232–2241, 1976.

79. Eagan RT, Frytak S, Creagan ET, *et al.*: Phase II study of cyclophosphamide, adriamycin and cis-dichlorodiammineplatinum by infusion in patients with adenocarcinoma and large cell carcinoma of the lung. Cancer Treat Rep 63:1589–1591, 1979.

80. Alberts P, Brunner K, Martz G, *et al.*: Treatment of bronchogenic carcinoma with simultaneous or sequential combination chemotherapy including methotrexate, cyclophosphamide, procarbazine and vincristine. Cancer 38:2208–2216, 1976.

81. Livingston RB, Fee WH, Einhorn LH, *et al.*: BACON (bleomycin, adriamycin, CCNU, oncovin and nitrogen mustard) in squamous cell lung cancer. Cancer 37:1237–1242, 1976.

82. Miller T, McMahon L, Livingston R: Extensive adenocarcinoma and large cell undifferentiated carcinoma of the lung treated with 5-FU, vincristine, and mitomycin-C (FOMi). Cancer Treat Rep 64:1241–1245, 1980.

83. Gralla RJ, Casper ES, Kelsen DP, *et al.*: Cisplatin and vindesine combination chemotherapy for advanced carcinoma of the lung: a randomized trial investigating two dosage schedules. Ann Intern Med 95:414–420, 1981.

84. Lad TE, Nelson RB, Diekamp D, *et al.*: Immediate *versus* postponed combination chemotherapy (CAMP) for unresectable non-small cell lung cancer: a randomized trial. Cancer Treat Rep 65:973–978, 1981.

85. Hyde L, Wolf J, McCracken S, *et al.*: Natural course of inoperable lung cancer. Chest 64:309–312, 1973.

86. Creech RH, Mehta CR, Cohen M, *et al.*: Results of a Phase II protocol for evaluation of new chemotherapeutic regimens in patients with inoperable non-small cell lung carcinoma (EST-2575, Generation I). Cancer Treat Rep 65: 431–438, 1981.

87. Livingston RB, Heilbrun L, Lehane D, *et al.*: Comparative trial of combination chemotherapy in extensive squamous carcinoma of the lung: A Southwest Oncology Group Study. Cancer Treat Rep 61:1632–1629, 1977.

88. Chahinian A, Arnold D, Cohen J, *et al.*: Chemotherapy for bronchogenic carcinoma. JAMA 237:2392–2396, 1977.

89. Vogl SE, Mehta CR, Cohen MH: MACC chemotherapy of adenocarcinoma and epidermoid carcinoma of the lung. Low response rate in a cooperative group study. Cancer 44:864–868, 1979.

90. Ruckdeschel JC, Mehta CR, Salazar OM, *et al.*: Chemotherapy for inoperable, non-small cell bronchogenic carcinoma: EST-2575, Generation II. Cancer Treat Rep 65:965–972, 1981.

91. Bitran JD, Desser RK, DeMeester TD, *et al.*: Metastatic non-oat cell bronchogenic carcinoma. Therapy with cyclophosphamide, doxorubicin, methotrexate, and procarbazine (CAMP). JAMA 240: 2743–2746, 1978.

92. Cambareri RJ, Smith FP, Macdonald JS, *et al.*: CAMP (cyclophosphamide, doxorubicin,

methotrexate, and procarbazine) for epidermoid and large cell anaplastic carcinoma of the lung. Cancer Treat Rep 65:317–320, 1981.

93. Ruckdeschel JC, Mehta CR, Salazar OM, *et al.*: Chemotherapy for metastatic non-small cell bronchogenic carcinoma: EST-2575, Generation III, HAM *versus* CAMP. Cancer Treat Rep 65:959–963, 1981.

94. Evans WK, Feld R, De Boer G, *et al.*: Cyclophosphamide, doxorubicin and cisplatin in the treatment of non-small cell bronchogenic carcinoma. Cancer Treat Rep 65:947–954, 1981.

95. Knost JH, Greco FA, Hande KR, *et al.*: Cyclophosphamide, doxorubicin, and cisplatin in the treatment of advanced non-small cell lung cancer. Cancer Treat Rep 65:941–945, 1981.

96. Robert F, Birch R, Krauss S, *et al.*: Randomized comparison of cyclophosphamide (C), adriamycin (A), methotrexate (M), and folinic acid (F) *vs* cyclosphamide, adriamycin and cis-platinum *vs* cyclophosphamide and adriamycin in advanced non-small cell lung cancer. Proc Am Soc Clin Oncol 22:503, 1981.

97. Davis S, Rambotti P, Park YK: Combination cyclophosphamide, doxorubicin, and cisplatin (CAP) chemotherapy for extensive non-small cell carcinomas of the lung. Cancer Treat Rep 65:955-958, 1981.

98. Langotte V, Thomas D, Holoye P, *et al.*: Bleomycin and 5-fluorouracil for non-oat cell bronchogenic carcinoma. Cancer Treat Rep 60:61–68, 1976.

99. Aisner J, Hansen HH: Commentary: Current status of chemotherapy for non-small cell lung cancer. Cancer Treat Rep 65:979–986, 1981.

100. Ruckdeschel J, Mehta C, Creech R: Chemotherapy of advanced non-oat cell carcinoma: The Eastern Cooperative Oncology Group Experience. In: Hansen HH, Dombernowsky P (eds). Abstracts II World Conference Abstracts II World Conference on Lung Cancer. Copenhagen: Excerpta Medica, 1980, p 237.

101. Vogelzang N, Bonomi P, Rossof A, *et al.*: Cyclophosphamide, adriamycin, methotrexate and procarbazine (CAMP) treatment of non-oat cell bronchogenic carcinoma. Cancer Treat Rep 62:1595–1597, 1978.

102. Livingston RB, Einhorn LH, Bodey GP, *et al.*: COMB (cyclophosphamide, oncovin, methyl-CCNU, and bleomycin). A four-drug combination in solid tumors. Cancer 36:-327–332, 1975.

103. Richards F, Cooper R, White D, *et al.*: Advanced epidermoid lung cancer – prolonged survival after chemotherapy. Cancer 46:34–37, 1980.

104. Vosika GJ: Large cell bronchogenic carcinoma – prolonged disease-free survival following chemotherapy. JAMA 241:594–595, 1979.

105. Shields TW, Humphrey EW, Eastridge CE, *et al.*: Adjuvant cancer chemotherapy after resection of carcinoma of the lung. Cancer 40:2057–2062, 1977.

106. Shields TW, Robinette CD, Keehn MS: Bronchial carcinoma treated by adjuvant cancer chemotherapy. Arch Surg 109:329–333, 1974.

107. Higgins GA, Shields TW: Experience of the Veterans Administration Surgical Adjuvant Group. Prog Cancer Res Therapy 11:433–442, 1979.

108. Stott H, Stephens RJ, Fox W, *et al.*: Five-year follow-up of cytoxic chemotherapy as an adjuvant to surgery in carcinoma of the bronchus. Br J Cancer 34: 167–173, 1976.

109. Legha S, Muggia F: Adjuvant chemotherapy in lung cancer. An appraisal of past studies. In: Progress in Cancer Research and Therapy: Lung Cancer. Muggia FM, Rozenzweig M (eds). New York, NY: Raven Press, Vol 11, 1979, p 405.

110. Sealy R: Combined radiotherapy and chemotherapy in non-small cell carcinoma of the lung. Prog Cancer Res Therapy 11:315–323, 1979.

111. Host H: Cyclophosphamide (NSC-26271) as an adjuvant to radiotherapy in the treatment

of unresectable bronchogenic carcinoma. Cancer Chemotherapy Rep 4:161–164, 1973.

112. Krant MJ, Chalmers TC, Dederick MM, *et al.*: Comparative trial of chemotherapy and radiotherapy in patients with nonresectable cancer of the lung. Am J Med 35:363–373, 1963.

113. Carr DT, Childs DS, Lee RE: Radiotherapy plus 5-FU compared to radiotherapy alone for inoperable and unresectable bronchogenic carcinoma. Cancer 29:375–380, 1972.

114. Takita H, Hollinshead AC, Rizzo DJ, *et al.*: Treatment of inoperable lung carcinoma: A combined modality approach. Ann Thoracic Surg 28:363–368, 1978.

INDEX